The
Gift
of a
Child

The
Gift
of a
Child

MARY ANN THOMPSON

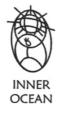

INNER
OCEAN

Inner Ocean Publishing, Inc.
P.O. Box 1239
Makawao, Maui, HI 96768-1239

Cover design: Bill Greaves
Cover photo: Stone
Interior photo: Nancy Bensley
Interior page design: Bill Greaves
Typography: Debra Lordan
Copy editor: Kirsten Whatley

Publisher Cataloging-in-Publication Data

Thompson, Mary Ann. The gift of a child / Mary Ann Thompson.
  --Makawao, HI : Inner Ocean, 2002.

       p. ; cm.
    ISBN 1-930722-17-6
       1. Thompson, Mary Ann. 2. Surrogate
    motherhood. 3. Surrogate motherhood--
    Psychological aspects. 4. Mother and child.
    5. Motherhood. I. Title.

HQ759.5 .T56 2002
306.8743--dc21   CIP

Printed in Canada by Friesens

9 8 7 6 5 4 3 2 1

To Alycia,
the mother of my daughter.

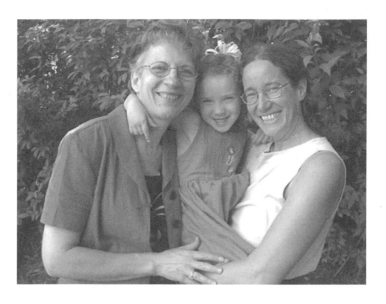

Mother's Day 2002

Contents

Acknowledgments

Gratitude erupts. The truth is that nothing I do is mine alone. These words came out of me because they were encouraged:

by Eden-Lee Murray whose open eyes and heart found my story, and Roger Jellinek whose insightful and sensitive editing suggestions made the story whole; together their believing in this book has made all the difference;

by all the others who are Inner Ocean for their skill, humanity, and zestful commitment to the right ideals: especially John Elder, Bill Greaves, John Nelson, Kirsten Whatley, and Debra Lordan.

by brave friends who read and critiqued the manuscript: Beth Cullen, Eileen Zimmerman, Ann Smith,

The Gift of a Child

Sandra Looney, Carol Peters;

by husband JD who gave me the space to work, who listened and read and helped me to remember, who walked the path beside me through this unusual adventure;

by friends who over the years encouraged me to write: especially Thomas Fassett, Char Reif, Shelly Matthews, and teachers David Downing and Tom Peek;

by the writers I have read, published and unpublished, whose courage outlasts their fear;

by the Mystery who gives both impulse and means;

to all these I extend my open-hearted thanks.

And finally to Mylah, who is by far more giver than gift: thank you, dear Bear Cub, for being born to us all and for teaching me so much in these first few years.

1
The Beginning of a Beginning

Inside the Great Mystery, we belong first and finally to ourselves.

I learned that lesson through the process of choosing to become a surrogate mother, through the pregnancy and birthing and separating, and through the ongoing experience of mother love at a great distance. Sometimes eagerly, other times reluctantly, I have learned to trust my life to that stark truth.

Four of us planned and entered into a pregnancy— two yearning to raise a child, two desiring the experience of pregnancy and birthing. We began as self-aware as people can be before such an unusual adventure. Each of us has ended up with more than we expected. More joy, more pain, more growth.

What was mine to learn rattled my bones and called

to remember the truth in the midst of unraveling, and the certainty that one can love with an open heart.

Perhaps the broader gift of this peculiar pregnancy and birth is that it reveals the slim filament that threads us together bead-to-bead across nation and race, across generation and circumstance: we each have been born. This story could be told for each of us. We found our way to birth. Peeled of the sentiment and the layers of external expectation, the raw truth is that we do find our own way. We do it. Inside the Mystery, we create ourselves.

Near the town of Copan Ruinas in Honduras is a small ruin several miles away from the main archeological site, where for hundreds of years Mayan women came to give birth. With the help of a guide, my husband and I visited this place. Power still echoes through the sparsely wooded ravine and its sweet-sounding brook.

As we approached the site, there were large stones engraved with symbols I did not understand. I touched them, tracing the design shapes. One oval obelisk was carved with a child emerging from a woman, the woman's mouth open, and the child's arms wildly extended. Two stones formed a doorway, one crudely shaped into a frog—a being of the water and the earth, and the other signed with a holy circle marked into quarters. Walking between them and turning uphill, I saw a natural hillside, a rocky meadow. To one side a twisted tree bloomed, whirring with bees. My husband and our guide walked toward its sparse shade.

Then I comprehended what I was looking at. In this place the rocks were shaped like powerful recliners, birthing stones, natural formations slightly shaped to provide hand and foot bracing places for the work of labor. I listened for the reverberating sounds of birth. I sat in the rock chairs. The proportions were exactly right! I didn't sit long. The power there was too great, and I was simply a spectator. I settled, crouching near the stones, touching the multicolored sand between the rocks, sand I knew had once been wet with sweat, sweet-smelling amniotic fluid, and sticky blood.

For how many women, how many children, for how many years was this place a doorway?

When any child is born, many are born. A father is born, he who a moment earlier was only a man. A mother is born, who for months had been merely a pregnant woman. A sister or brother is born, who was just a child before. And beyond that: cousins, aunts, grandparents, perhaps the whole world is changed by one moment of emergence, that draining out of water and drawing in of breath. She is born, and we are born too, changed by the startling, wavering announcement of life, of autonomy, of existence.

On my forty-first birthday, March 15, 1998, I conceived of the idea of becoming pregnant with a child my friends would raise. Birthdays are a time of reflection for me. I was thinking about my friends Alycia and Mandel. They lived in a small town in Wisconsin. I had known Alycia for twenty years. They loved each other. They were hard-working, good people. For many years they had a sadness, a sorrow, an unresolved tension in their lives. They wanted to be parents.

They had given up on conceiving a child of their own after many years of trying. Medical tests had revealed Mandel's sperm was viable and Alycia did ovulate although not regularly. They tried as many procedures and options as they could afford, and there was no pregnancy. There was a brief possibility of an adoption that February, a possibility that came to them unbidden, awakening again their desire to be a family. But, once again, seemingly for the last time, the situation was insurmountable and their lives moved on.

I reflected about the pain of hope. The cost and effort of hope. The powerful willing of the soul to imagine a good thing that never comes. I had recently finished working in my profession, and had a year and a half of time before my husband would retire from teaching physics at a liberal arts college. What would fill that year? What project, what task? I first thought of raising money for Alycia and Mandel to help them pursue adoption if they still wanted to do that. But they were both in their early forties. There was no certainty that adoption would be possible.

From the time I was a child myself I wanted to experience pregnancy and birthing. If my body was made to do something so rich and strong, then I wanted the experience. If one has legs, one wants to run. It was just like that for me. The procreative mystery was around me, beguiling me. Our neighbor had an almost yearly swollen belly. I felt both interested to the point of staring, and embarrassed for thinking about what I was seeing.

As a child and teen, pregnancy and birth had the same allure for me that sex did. My sisters and I had a plastic model of a woman with transparent skin and removable organs that fit together like puzzle pieces. She came with two options: regular and pregnant. I held the fetus, housed it in the clear eggshell uterus, and wedged it in her body, replacing the regular intestines with the oddly arched pregnant intestines. Replacing the flat-bellied front with the alternative, a voluptuous full-bellied one, she was transformed. What wonder!

So powerful were those experiences and desires that all these years later, the idea of my having a child wasn't far away. Now I had time, desire, and courage. It would take courage, great courage. What if I had a child, if we all had a child together? What if I could experience this thrilling process I had for years looked in at, my nose to its window? What if Alycia and Mandel's fervent hope could be realized?

Many nights during the years of Alycia's infertility I had dreamed of her holding a baby. I saw a child and the joy on my friend's face. I had told her of those dreams, hesitating to add their promise to her failing endurance. What if I were to be a part of how those dreams took flesh? Suddenly, my body was a flute being played: waves of sound and breath moving through me.

I talked with my husband, JD. He was sitting right beside me. We were working on a computer project together as this idea burst like a sprouting seed. I asked him what he thought about the idea. I asked him what it would be like for him to have me carry a child that was genetically unrelated to him. We talked. We considered. Our conversation included how the demands of pregnancy, especially at forty-one, and the unknown experience of being a "surrogate" mother might affect our marriage. Our early apprehensions quickly dissolved in JD's vigorous support and encouragement.

I called my sister to test my idea. In her gentle wisdom she was realistically cautious. I heard the subtle shades of hesitation in her voice. The idea was such a surprise that she withheld saying much. At the same time, she was clearly supportive of any decision I would make. I felt excited explaining the idea to her, a little fearful of her realism. Ideas appear so different outside of one's head. This proposal, now shared twice, was wanting to grow.

So I called Alycia, my friend of twenty years, a woman brave and tenacious. A woman aware of life's complexities, she was skilled in exploring the deep emotions and questions. She had lived through many painful experiences and emerged still swimming, nose above the water. I said, as gently as I could into the hum of a phone wire, "How about if we all make a baby for you? My egg, Mandel's sperm. My pregnancy, your child?"

She was silent. She cried softly. She didn't say much. I remember the quiet joy and the fear we both had of hope reemerging, hope for a child for her to hold and kiss. There is an exquisite torture in hope. She hung up to talk with her husband, to explain the tears in her voice to him.

Mandel is a gentle man, with a genuine, quiet soul. He loves his parents and has lived most of his life close to home. The first thing I heard about him was the story Alycia told me: A young bird had fallen from its nest. Mandel went to investigate and reached toward the tiny nestling. It jumped up onto his finger. As he spoke to it, it fell asleep in the curl of his big hand, and nestled there long enough for Alycia to go get her camera and photograph them. He hunts, too, to provide venison that they eat. He drives trucks for a living. He has a smile that sparkles. He would now have many thoughts to sift through with his strong hands, his quiet spirit.

Alycia called me back later that evening and said, "Yes, let's keep thinking about it." Yes, she said. Mandel had said yes. JD said yes. And so four yeses were planted on that day, my birthday. In the weeks ahead, either they would grow into certainty or die from doubt and fear. Four brave and tiny yeses. A first birth. The beginning of a beginning.

2 Gestating the Idea

Alycia and I talked. Many phone calls of talk. I asked how she would feel raising a child who ran around her living room wearing my face. What if this baby looked like me? How would that continual reminder wear? Alycia didn't see raising a child who was obviously genetically tied elsewhere to be a problem. She had been interested in adopting and didn't have the need Mandel did of having a genetic tie with a child. Her child would be her child.

We spoke of every detail we could imagine. What if the experiment didn't work and there was no child, would we still want to have tried? What if our friendship were compromised by the huge unknowns we were considering? We turned every stone and explored what we found underneath. We didn't have answers for all of our questions, but nothing seemed to block the way ahead.

We had such easy rapport and agreement about the details of the arrangement. We talked about who would name the baby; Alycia and Mandel would without question. We fantasized about the birth and spending the baby's first gentle week together, so Baby could nurse, making the transition slow and loving for us all.

How would I deal with it, that inevitable time of separation? All I knew was that I didn't know. I had experienced loss: dear and precious parts of myself; and central figures in my life, loves that did not ripen. I had moved many times. I had honestly loved people in my work and then cut ties. I knew loss and leaving and being left. I told Alycia I believed I could live through the separation.

My sister, Laura Jean, a neonatal intensive care nurse, was invaluable. We talked about what risks there were for me. At forty-one, was I too old? Not at all she said, although bearing the stresses and the recovery might be harder for me now. I asked, was there a risk from old eggs? Yes, there was a greater risk for abnormalities. We wondered how it would be to attempt conception through insemination. Would it be embarrassing; would it seem unnatural? Laura Jean asked how I would feel if I didn't get pregnant, which I had only superficially considered. She knew it was not only possible but probable. (After I was pregnant she told me we had a one-in-ten chance at each insemination at my age.)

I asked my sister how it felt to be pregnant, how hard it was to recover from birthing, what effect my asthma might have on a pregnancy and in labor. She helped me explore my questions, offering information, wisdom, and most powerfully openness. Her knowledge was important. Her love was precious.

And she asked the question that came to me so many times: How will that moment be when the baby leaves with her mom and dad, and I am left behind? I answered, confident and sure, that it would just be a hard moment in a wonderful experience. Somehow I would incorporate the hurt into the whole.

My sister walks a tightrope with ease, a tightrope of loving but not influencing. She was afraid for the hurt I would feel, the pain of loss so inevitable in this venture. She knew about the strength of those ties that would need to be loosened and released. Yet she joined my exuberance at the prospect of pregnancy, the possibility of experiencing this marvel my body was made to do.

As I considered the idea personally, I was thrilled with the thought of being filled with child, of being strong and powerful in this amazing way, thrilled by the possibility that I could be included, that my genes would go on into the future. But, more than that, I would know what others meant when they talked of birth, of pregnancy, of the love that exists only in the parent-child bond. I wanted to be inside that room I had looked into through the window. In that room the adults had children. Many my age had grandchildren. I was eager for what seemed out of reach, eager to know myself in this basic way, as a mother, as a life giver.

Once, when I was six or seven, I peeked around the corner of my auntie's bedroom to see my cousin lying on her bed nursing her baby. She welcomed me in. Watching her was terrific. The room was filled with a loving warmth: the wet sounds of baby sucking and the soft contentment sounds, the look of confidence and pride in my cousin's eyes. She was connected to the world in the same way the child was connected to her. The circuit was full of power.

I was fascinated about the whole process of birth and of babies. Yet for most of my childbearing years, being single, being filled with my own agenda and with the refuse of childhood trauma, I didn't want to raise a child. I didn't want to be responsible for another human being for a long time. I knew that I needed all of me.

Then, when I was finally ready to, I thought about becoming pregnant through donor insemination and raising a child as a single mom. I was finally ready to commit to another human being. I was ready to welcome another into my life. At the time I was a single United Methodist minister. It would have been difficult as a pastor in a small rural town to choose to become a single mother. Just as I was planning to begin the process of telling my intentions to the two churches for which I was pastor, the denominational officials, and my family, I met a man who changed everything.

JD and I met through a mutual friend. His friend and I were at a meeting in his town. We decided to all go to dinner together. We enjoyed Thai food and a slide show about the rain forest, and were joined by his brother for tea at JD's home after that. I noticed JD's open heart, his love of adventure, the warm respectful way he related to our mutual friend. His home was full of painting and sculpture and music, and yet unpretentious. I watched his hands express his words as we talked about the rain forests, an upcoming trip he would be making to attend a physics conference, the side trips for white water rafting and sea kayaking. All this from one who grew up a South Dakota farm boy. After spending a wonderful evening talking and trading stories with him, the thought came unbidden as I walked away from his front door: If I can connect with another adult like that, I don't need to have a baby.

First that thought, then the fear, like a damp chilling wind, fear that was the shadow of feeling at home with a man I barely knew, fear about the depth of my initial connection with him. What was I thinking, being that honest?

At thirty-eight, I had never been in a long-term partnership. I had had several relationships over the years—few serious ones, most of those across many miles or other great distances. In the previous years I had met several people in whom I was interested. None of them were interested in a relationship with me.

These multiple rejections made me wary of the feeling of attraction. Would this meeting end in more embarrassment and rejection? I did not want to endure it again. But how could I not try, how could I not open again to a sunrise when my soul so craved that warmth and light?

My plans for becoming a single mother were eclipsed by JD's presence in my life. We talked on the phone after a few days. It was clear there were two people in this same wonderful, fearful place. The tender place. The magic place of love's birth.

I believe in resurrection in this way: There are moments where life chooses us. We can often, then, choose life again, choose life in spite of the painful risks and all the death and darkness around us.

Over the next months, I shivered from the fear and made the steps to test my trust in myself. Could I trust my feelings, my intuitions? Could I believe my sense of the relationship progressing between us? We are in any moment the products of our pasts—resurrection or no resurrection—and the questioning threatened much of my faith. At the same time, courage seeped in like an underground spring. I crossed the bridge of connection. A friendship was formed, a dance, a way of moving through time together. First we made friendship, then we made love, now we were making marriage, step-by-step.

JD and I were clear that we wouldn't be starting a family of our own: He had grown children and young grandchildren. I didn't want both a marriage and a child. We each wanted a life for the two of us. We thought sometimes, in a romantic way, what children we created might be like. But clearly we wanted our time to be for other things. There was never any doubt or conflict about having children.

Out of this new way of life, I felt more and more of myself emerging; more of my life seemed to be mine. Within the context of this new stability and tranquility, my desire to experience pregnancy and birth had a less desperate quality. When the thought of being a surrogate mother came to me in the context of my marriage, it seemed more an option than something I was compelled to do or be. It took more than two feet on the ground in my life to take on this task; it took four, mine and JD's.

In the days following my birthday, JD and I talked about the possibility of my carrying a child. We were excited that I might explore a childhood dream, that I might experience this wonderful part of life, and that he and I would share such holy time together. It fit into our life right then, with my being unemployed and him approaching retirement. What a gift this might be to us.

Alycia and I had met while attending theological seminary. We met on a stairway. Alycia was coming downstairs with her parents, both of whom were missionaries in Brazil now enrolling in an academic time of renewal. She was starting her graduate study as well. Al Caldwell, the seminary librarian, was showing these three new students around the school. I was starting my second year. Because I worked in the library, and because my mother had preceded me in seminary by two years, Al and I had often talked about the unique gifts and frustrations of sharing graduate school with a parent. Al made a connection between Alycia and me with our similar circumstance and introduced us.

What I remember of the encounter is that our eyes connected. They locked. We seemed to see far into each other. There was disclosure beyond words. It was a moment when I knew something important was happening.

We became friends. In our final year of seminary we even shared an apartment with another friend. I enjoyed Alycia's bilingual brain (she had grown up in Brazil speaking English and Portuguese), her diverse experience, her courage. One summer she traveled with a group to Israel to participate in an archeological dig and visited Greece. There, she spent time with some people she knew and took a trip out to the islands by herself. I admired that independence. She was a distance runner, thin and strong. She smoked cigarettes to defy her strict upbringing—a small rebellion against parents she clearly loved and respected.

That last year of school, we both dated men who weren't good mates for us. The four of us were together often. Looking back I see that the affinity wasn't between the pairs, but was between Alycia and me. I loved her. She was not my only friend then, perhaps not even my best friend in the sense that others shared more of my growth in thinking and evolving in those years. But, for better or worse, Alycia and I were like sisters.

She was the only one from school with whom I kept in contact over the years. We shared the end of her first marriage, talking endlessly over the weekend before she decided it was over. At that wedding I had watched her greet her cousin Mandel. She brightened in his presence. I asked that day if she was marrying the right man. Years later she did marry Mandel. They struggled with the social mores. They agonized about the family tensions their relationship created. But their love, and their desire to be together, won.

After graduate school, our friendship continued,

mostly by phone, as we grew through parallel early experiences as new pastors in rural midwestern towns. We both had other friends who shared our lives in more intimate ways. But Alycia and I did keep in touch.

We talked about anything. She had a great desire to have a child. As a girl, she had been told by a physician that conceiving would likely be difficult for her. We joked during those years that I could conceive and birth a child for her. When Alycia and Mandel worked through the social stigma of being married cousins and satisfied themselves that the genetic risks of their having a child together were not too serious, they went off birth control and waited for the magic moment to come.

They waited; their attention would peak as each month went by. Then they waited like people whose bus was always late, overtly frustrated, making jokes to cover the anger. Eventually they waited like parents whose child was way too late. They knotted up, their faces were clouded over and they thought the worst.

The medical community could offer little. Many procedures were too expensive for them. Some tests were inconclusive. They did what they could. Alycia took medicine to force her ovaries to produce eggs. They turned their lovemaking into a contest to win a prize. Months and years. Months and years. The magic moment didn't happen.

They came to some acceptance of their childlessness

the summer before I suggested we try surrogacy. That fall, the timbre of Alycia's voice changed. She began moving on with her life. In winter there was a trip back to Brazil to visit her parents. A baby in a neighboring village was in need of parents. For a whole weekend they thought they had a son. Both Alycia and Mandel grew attached to the idea. On Monday, desperate calls were made to the governmental offices who could help them accomplish this thing. The Brazilian officials could have the papers ready in a matter of a week or two. The U.S. officials said it would take a year's time and about twenty thousand dollars to have the documents to adopt and bring that child home. The cost and the wait made the possibility impossible for them.

When she told me this story, her desire was so strong and her avenues so exhausted, that I felt I had to act. Twenty years after we had met on a stairway, Alycia and I were looking into this other possibility, and we were again looking full into each other's eyes to see what truth was there.

JD and I were trying to balance our idealism with some practicality. We met with an attorney to discuss the legal ramifications of surrogacy for us. Surrogacy is governed by state laws. She knew of a situation the previous decade where a woman in South Dakota had been a gestational surrogate for the embryo of her daughter and son-in-law. She knew of no other people in South Dakota who had been or were exploring being surrogates of any kind. She was intrigued and curious, and saw problems, legal and otherwise. We sat with her as she raised issues: What if the child was born with disabilities, who paid the medical bills? What if I was injured by this? What if we needed the court to take action, how difficult and expensive would that be? She strongly recommended a detailed legal contract be written and signed, although she doubted it would be enforceable because the two couples lived in different states. Drawing up a legal contract would take many months. We appreciated her objective view of the hazards out there in the mist of the future.

I searched the Internet and found agencies that "broker" surrogacy. They listed their criteria for surrogate mothers, and I did not meet them. I was too old. And I did not meet the requirement that a surrogate already have children of her own in order to give informed consent. I read many stories on websites from parents whose children were born from surrogates, and a few stories written by surrogate moms. The tales were poignant, not too edited, very expressive. I was astonished to see the variety of experiences through which people were going. Many situations were far different from ours, but a few were similar. The emotions were there to see. I looked at contracts used to define the relationships among the participants. I feasted on the descriptions, the evidence that our idea of surrogacy could work.

I learned that what we were planning to do was illegal in several states. It angered me that legislators could make something so private unlawful. I understood the dangers of selling babies, of using poor women as baby-making machines, of women of means not choosing to have the inconvenience of pregnancy and hiring it out like one might send out the laundry. But we were not doing any of that. What power did they think they had to control the choices we were considering?

Our thoughts grew more informed, if not expert, and our opinions evolved. JD and I felt that unless the decisions were based on trust in ourselves, we would not be able to proceed. Our rights would not be protected by anything other than trust. Legal systems would not protect us. Alycia and Mandel's promises would not protect us. We had to make a decision we knew to be right inside our own bones.

What is trustworthy for me in such situations is the deepest place inside me. In that place, largely without words, my decision remained firm and strong. I considered the legal ramifications, the possible unromantic side effects, the problems that could emerge. It was essential to consider it all. And in the quiet of my heart, in the place where I stand when everything else is blown away from me, my decision was unwavering.

Another significant issue was facing us as a couple. JD had prostate cancer. He found the cancer in a very early stage four months before we considered surrogacy. We cried when we found out, screamed and yelled at the implications for our life together. We then settled into finding options for his treatment. He chose Brachytherapy—the implantation of radioactive seeds into his prostate to kill the cancer.

We chose an excellent doctor in Seattle to do the procedure and flew there in early February to meet with him. JD was accepted into their program. In mid-February he began a treatment of hormone therapy to shrink his prostate. The treatment virtually eliminated his testosterone, which both controlled the cancer and shrunk his prostate. The hormone therapy was done so it would be possible, later in June, to implant the seeds.

So, as we moved through the process of considering this life-making adventure, JD and I did it in the context of the word "cancer." Prostate cancer is usually slow growing, and JD's was a moderately aggressive form. There was no rational reason to think that death was around the corner for him, but cancer easily conjures images of struggle and pain and death. For us, those images had faces of people we had loved.

We wondered about the wisdom of mixing pregnancy with prostate cancer. But at that point his situation seemed on a path that was going well, and he was generally symptom free. From all we had learned, his most difficult time would be July and August, one and two months after the seeds were implanted. Each of us decided we could do these two life-changing things at the same time.

Alycia and I talked again on the phone. During the conversation I realized I wouldn't feel right about being pregnant unless she was the one who inseminated me. Something about having her husband's sperm inside of me was unnerving if it weren't happening by her own direct action. We began to question the need of having medical professionals involved in the insemination at all. The four of us knew what was needed. There are many resources telling women how to do their own donor inseminations. JD grew up on a farm: He said he knew the process. It seemed that we didn't need anything more than what we could do for each other, and so we decided to try inseminating on our own.

I thought about the risk to me of HIV/AIDS. I talked to Alycia about it. Trusting takes on gravity in moments like that. I had to judge if Alycia and Mandel would have shared honestly with each other, let alone with me, the risky behaviors that could have exposed either of them to HIV. To insist on a test is standard procedure in the surrogacy agencies. Sperm banks protect their clients by testing samples again six months after the donation and only then release the frozen sperm.

Alycia knew of no HIV risk from either of them. I didn't doubt their answers and believed they wouldn't knowingly endanger me.

Was I foolish not to ask for them to be tested? I decided their words were enough. Trusting is a web built bit by bit. If we were going to move ahead, there would be no way to take out the risk for any of us. We were all risking our lives. In the still place, I still said yes.

I talked with Alycia, saying I knew I would need expressions of support from them—cards, notes, phone calls and such. I needed to have continuing assurance she and Mandel were supporting me and with me through this time. She assured me she understood.

While talking with JD, I unearthed a fear: What if they backed out mid-pregnancy? What if they conceived by themselves, and didn't want some variation of "twins?" It happens. Sometimes a couple not able to conceive gets pregnant soon after their adoptive child arrives. Like priming a pump. To purposely conceive, knowing I didn't want to raise a child, is a strange choice to make. Would JD help me through the difficult decisions if Alycia and Mandel backed out of our agreement? Was he willing to proceed not knowing how all those variables would work out? He was.

It is amazing to wander through such complexity. There are many variables, many emotions, many physical factors. There is no way to know what will happen for certain. And still, for all the big decisions in our lives—for anyone making a choice to have a baby, or to marry, or to enter into an intimate relationship, or to do some particularly potent thing—there are layers and layers of unknown. Clarity comes, not from exhausting all the variables and testing all the possibilities in controlled circumstances; clarity and certainty come from deeper in our awareness.

Wandering through this decision-making process was like learning to ride a bicycle; with all the complex instructions and the skills of balance and coordination mastered, finally you just "get it" and take off. Suddenly it is time and you choose.

3 The Conception

The worries seemed to work themselves out. After a few intensive weeks of inviting all the possible problems to surface, the four of us were still ready to move ahead. So I checked my body cycles with a calendar and guessed when my next time of ovulation would be—the weekend of April 9. We decided to plan toward the first of four possible monthly cycles of inseminations.

The chosen date was a full moon, which I loved. It was also Easter weekend, which also seemed marvelously appropriate. We planned a visit to Wisconsin, where Alycia and Mandel lived. Their work schedules made it easier for us to drive to them, and so we did.

The week before we went, I bought some ovulation predictor kits, to add some science to the process. Somehow it seemed like a clandestine thing to have in my shopping cart. I snaked through the store toward the checkout, eyes low, hoping not to see anyone I knew. The box glowed in neon.

Women are valued for their fertility. In my forty-one years I had internalized many messages of being unworthy because I had chosen to be child free. How dare I now venture into the realm of the *real* women. But I did dare. I awkwardly bought the kit. A few days before the trip I began to test myself, just to be sure that I didn't ovulate early. Everything was working.

One of those days just before the planned weekend, JD said to me that I could go alone if I wanted to, that he didn't need to go. A chill went through me. Maybe he wasn't as "into" this as he had been saying. I shared my feelings, and we cried and talked. He was feeling as if he wasn't needed.

How startling! I needed him so. He was essential to this process. In that moment I knew it was just as important for him to be physically involved in the insemination process as Alycia, and that if he wasn't, I didn't feel I could go ahead. He smiled. He decided to come.

JD was teaching until noon on Friday. I thought I would be ovulating on Saturday. He had to be back home on Monday evening. That didn't leave much of a window for my body to be unpredictable. I felt a strange pressure to perform: So many lives were circling around my cycle; so many people looking to my rhythm for a dance beat.

Alycia's parents were visiting for the holiday, so this event was to take place in the midst of extended family. I wished it weren't so, but I wanted to proceed anyway. We were only going to have four tries at conceiving before the birthing would conflict with JD's time of retirement, and I was ready to try.

Driving to Wisconsin on Friday, we alternated between talking and silence. It was good to be together. We made a list of issues to discuss with Alycia and Mandel, listening to ourselves and each other as honestly as we could. Our decision to invite new life on a full moon and on Easter weekend brought us great delight.

We arrived after supper. Alycia and I hugged. Mandel and I glanced at each other—I felt shy and excited observing him with completely new eyes. A friend had asked me how Mandel looked, wanting to imagine how a child of our genes would appear. Now I looked at him with that question in my head. I quickly focused back on JD. We all were smiling, maybe with more joy than with nervousness. Maybe.

Alycia's parents were introduced to JD. We all talked a little while but, though fully informed, they didn't seem comfortable with what we were about to do, instead: How was the drive? Nice to see the weather so warm! And Alycia's parents excused themselves to the guestroom. Alycia, Mandel, JD, and I settled into a comfortable quiet around the kitchen table. All really important things happen around such tables.

Mandel looked exhausted from a long day of hard work driving a truck for the landscaping company. We decided to talk things through the next day. And we knew we needed to make the most of this weekend. "Is there anything that would mean we wouldn't move ahead?" I asked. Each one in turn said no. We were ready.

So we decided to do an insemination that night. Mandel went off to the bathroom and Alycia showed us to their bedroom, where we would sleep. We walked back to the dining room. Alycia went back up to get some clothes from their bedroom for the next day. She came back in a while with a small jar tucked under her arm and said Mandel was done and they were ready. We showed her the small syringe we had brought along.

I had a shy moment, turned to JD, and snuggled myself into his arms. I felt the enormity of what was to come. I felt the embarrassment of having three sets of eyes focused on my very private self. I felt the strength of my wanting to do this, and I said, "Let's go." JD's eyes looked full of love and sweet support as I searched them one last time, looking for fear or reluctance.

In the bedroom I took off the necessary clothes and

lay down on the water bed. I asked JD to sit by me, and he settled in on my left side. Alycia sat beside me on the right. Mandel sat beside the bed, where he could see. There was a feeling of solemn power in that room. I breathed deeply and tried to just be there, in that moment that held such consequence. Calmness mixed with the excitement, and a profound intimacy formed among the four of us. Tranquility held us. It was a moment like none I've known.

Alycia looked at me holding the jar of Mandel's ejaculate. Her eyes were open wide, deep, and clear. "Are you sure?" she said to me. She was strong.

"Yes," I responded, sure, calm. I smiled. Her hands shook a little. We all laughed. "Don't spill it! Mandel is tired, remember?!"

I opened my legs and JD opened me for the syringe. Alycia asked if it hurt. No, I told her, everything was fine. JD held Alycia's hand and she filled me with the gift of her husband. It was done. We were flooded with emotion. Unnamed emotion. The kind that runs in rivers down faces and flies like a bird in the chest. We had an unceremonious moment as Mandel brought the pillow they had used for years to prop up Alycia's hips when they were trying to conceive. Together they put the pillow under me.

I looked up into three faces shining with love. I opened my arms and all three fell in. We lay laughing and crying, touching hands, lightly kissing our partners. Quiet words were exchanged by twos all around. The room was washed in the relief of tension broken. We stayed all together for the thirty minutes recommended to maximize our chances of conceiving. Someone invited the soul that wanted to come join this family to enter the process. We each added our words of invitation.

We laughed as Alycia put her hand on my tummy and pressed a little to sense and say what words could not. I said, "Don't push, Alycia, pull!" And we imagined my body welcoming the swimmers into me.

When Alycia and Mandel left to sleep on the living room hide-a-bed, JD got into bed beside me and I turned to him. I suddenly felt terrified and mixed up. I asked him how he felt. He was fine. I told him my feelings. I felt odd, as if I had betrayed him, as if I had done something wrong. He talked with me softly, saying he was fine, he was proud of me, he loved me. He is truly a remarkable man. My emotions passed through me and were gone.

Fears seem powerful when they are resisted, and yet exposed to the light of truth, they dissolve into manageable wisps of darkness. The holiness of that night, the sacred spirit, surrounded me again as it had during the insemination, like the sound of a drum beating strong. We slept.

Morning came, and the house was filled with movement and talk. It was an odd assortment of personalities that didn't fit very comfortably into a small house. Alycia and Mandel had to go to work. JD and I went for a day trip to a nearby nature preserve and listened to geese, looked for a small herd of bison living there, and drove a winding road among some tall trees.

We decided to walk. Having brought supplies for a picnic, we found a spot out of the relentless wind where the sunshine was bright through the thin, leafless branches. It was glorious! That time nourished us, reinforced us.

I did the ovulation test, and it was strongly positive, indicating that I would ovulate within the next few hours. Perfect timing! I reveled in my trustworthy body and the amazing perfection of this weekend. We had a long, luxurious time together under those trees.

Later that day, everyone had returned to Alycia and Mandel's house. JD and I had noticed the discomfort of Alycia's parents the night before and asked Alycia and Mandel if it would be appropriate to offer to talk with them. They appreciated our sensitivity and agreed it would be a good thing.

We approached the older couple, saying we had sensed their nervousness and the awkwardness of this situation for them. We offered to simply answer any of their questions and hear their concerns. They were understandably uneasy, not really sure about this thing we were doing. As they talked, they expressed it was fear for their daughter, Alycia; that her hopes would be raised and broken again. They worried I would change my mind about raising the child if we were able to conceive. They were fearful, yet properly supportive, and understood that this decision was not up to them. It was uncomfortable to listen to them. And it was important.

After they had expressed themselves, I shared my fear that Alycia and Mandel might change their minds midstream. Alycia's parents were shocked, saying, "They would never do that!"

And I said, "Likely not, but I am still afraid of it. As sure as you are that they will not break their word to me, I am sure I will not break faith with them either. I know that my assurance doesn't make you less afraid. I love Alycia, she is my friend, and I wouldn't hurt her. I can't imagine, loving her as her parents, how you must fear for her risking in this way."

JD tried, too, to assure them. Sharing information seemed to be the only real way to soften the tensions. I'm certain they worried every day—and maybe still do—that somehow I will change my mind. The books and TV movies consistently portray birth mothers refusing to honor their agreements to part with their children. Alycia's parents' path through the pregnancy and birth time must have been thorny as well as sweet.

There certainly were not any guarantees, for anyone.

I began to be aware of the number of people's lives who were drawn into this pursuit, into the potential tangle of miraculous gifts and serious pain. I expected Alycia's parents to see me as a way their prayers were being answered. Instead, it seemed I was perceived as bringing more risk. The suspicion was appreciable. I was surprised.

I knew why I was doing this astonishing thing, but others had a hard time comprehending why. My motives were clear and simple to me: I wanted selfishly to experience this wondrous process and secondarily to help my friends' dreams come true. But people don't knowingly choose hard things. And we all knew that the four of us making a baby together would be a difficult, rugged course for a long, long time to come.

Later on, I used that language often to tell people why I was doing surrogacy. I would explain all my reasons—selfish and altruistic—and then say, "People can choose hard things." Often this brought considerable conversation. We take the easy path as a general reaction to overstimulated and stressful lives. But often, the difficult path is richer and produces greater opportunity for growth and discovery.

That evening we did another insemination: This time the mood was joyful. The three of us waited in position for Mandel to join us. When he came into the bedroom, JD laughed and said, "Here comes Santa Claus!"

Just before Alycia inseminated me the second time, I felt the air shiver over my belly. It was a strange feeling, and I stopped the current process to describe what I felt. "I think we just made a baby!" And each of us responded with excitement and reluctance; almost believing, almost not believing that we could be really accomplishing this. I truly believe the first insemination was all we would have needed. I think the egg and sperm met right then, as the four of us were gathered in love. But, we proceeded with the second insemination as planned. The procedure was as flawless as before.

We did a third insemination on April 11, Easter Sunday morning. Again, this time was spirited, a time of loving and great anticipation. We were trying to temper our hope, but true hope is hard to reign in. Joy and years of realistic experience were both with us. We were courageous all together. Why would anyone try conceiving with less than four people?! It seemed to take that many hearts and hands to hold all the emotion.

JD and I packed up after Alycia, Mandel, and her parents went off to church. We drove home wondering if . . . wondering, could we just have . . . ? What an Easter! What a resurrection of hope in the possibilities of new life!

The first few days back home I was intensely self-aware. Testing my self for any twinges, any new feelings, any perception of being pregnant. I felt nothing new. Days went by, a week of days. Everything seemed ordinary.

I tried remembering that succeeding on the first try would be unusual. It often takes six cycles of donor inseminating for it to work. I tried to prepare myself for whatever the outcome—positive or negative.

But my excitement level was high, and it was hard to believe the magical weekend would not have been successful. Talking with Alycia was hard those days. She had been through hope deferred so many times and cautioned me. But hope is not cautious. And I felt her hoping, too.

One morning, as JD and I were out for our morning walk to check our gardens, I had a strange wave of weakness pass through me. Later I felt—or did I imagine I felt?—tenderness in my breasts. I had such high hopes that every possible sensation was mined for meaning. Many of the signs were similar between approaching menstruation and pregnancy. I just didn't know.

Our agreement was to do the pregnancy test while talking on the phone two weeks following the inseminations. I called Alycia Saturday night to see when would be a good time for us to do the test the next day. She said, "Let's just do it now!"

My heart was a drum. I got the kit. I tried to breathe. JD talked to Alycia on the phone as I went into the bathroom. Alycia's watch was our timer. We had to wait five minutes to see the results. I got too excited and went to see after only three minutes, and there was an unmistakable positive line. We screamed. We kissed our spouses. We hung up the phone to celebrate, promising to talk again in a few minutes. It was true: We had conceived! Four people had made a baby!

4

The First Trimester

The fears began to leach through the joy right away. I was at the top of the chairlift, and I was dumped off onto the fast snow, never having skied! I looked at my eyes in the mirror, self-consciously at first, and then again, later, deeply—was I the same? Was I in some way completely different? When no one was looking, I touched my belly, no different under my hand, but completely different.

One morning I made my ritual cup of holy coffee, the same cup as always, the same Sumatra whole beans, the same unbleached filter. It tasted bad. Coffee! It tasted bad! My self-image warped as the next few mornings the same thing happened. It wasn't my eyes that gave me away. I wasn't changed in a romantic way, but in a painfully pragmatic one! It wasn't that I knew it would be better if I didn't drink it or that I decided not to have coffee for the good of the pregnancy. It tasted repulsive, even vile. This wasn't about my being a hero and sacrificing for the baby. This bundle of cells had taken over, rearranging my taste buds and my identity. I slid off my own known path. The mountaintop tilted down and away, and the journey now begun didn't allow much choice. I pointed the tips of my skis downhill and let gravity take me. I had welcomed the first mild, occasional nausea that came, giggling with its confirmation that I was pregnant. But to have my taste for coffee leave: How could this little zygote do that? I was preparing for a romantic pregnancy, a Mona Lisa smile of a pregnancy, and the coffee ordeal just didn't fit. It was the first of many lessons.

The first trimester was something that mostly happened in my mind. I adapted my thinking. I wanted my preconceptions, my romantic scripts to be the way it really happened. Over and over I found that what I expected wasn't even close to what it was actually like to be pregnant. The actual experience usually brought even more growth and an even larger experience.

We had a friend over for dinner who teaches biology at the same college where my husband taught physics. In the course of the evening, we told him the adventure we were on. He talked with us about embryology and what might be happening developmentally on that very day for the new life in me: A ball of cells tumbling down the slope of my fallopian tubes, would be hollowing itself out, forming groups of cells to become a placenta, a body.

Who was deciding which cell would do what? Where was the guidance? I listened to all the details that had to go just right for implantation to occur and later for the major organ systems to form correctly. I could do little to affect the process. I was thinking I would somehow have a huge role to play. I hadn't known the placenta was the baby's making. I thought it was made by me to nourish the baby. In truth, it fended for itself.

I wasn't a nurturing, magical creator, I was the person who stocked the grocery shelves. It was a radical change in job perception. I was sitting in the bleachers, and the main show was going on inside my body with a new little actor-director calling almost all the shots!

I was anxious to find a health care provider for myself. As a generally healthy person, being pregnant didn't sound like a disease or a medical issue. I know a professional's training and background can greatly affect what she or he sees. I wanted a wellness perspective to guide this wonderful time in my life. We didn't need a clinic to achieve this pregnancy. I wanted health care but not rigid formulas and rules written to benefit the provider more than the pregnant woman. I didn't want or intend to release the reins of my experience to anyone else.

I know that often the medical community assumes one is "under" their care, and they make the decisions. If I need that, that is fine. But as long as I am healthy I don't want to submit to that treatment and routine. I wanted a guide, not a leader. I wanted support, not external control. I clearly wanted a midwife.

Looking in the phone book, I found the only midwife in town. I called and made an appointment with Teresa, hoping for someone who could work with me. When the day arrived, JD and I went in and sat in the room full of young women in various stages of pregnancy and older women we could only guess about. We were giddy. My name was called. The two of us went back to a little station in the labyrinth of hallways and rooms.

A nurse began asking me questions and filling out forms. She asked the date of my last period, and I said I could tell her the conception date. She smiled in condescension, "No, we figure things another way." She asked for some general information from me. Then she asked JD for his blood type.

He said, "That isn't relevant. I'm not the father."

"But you are her husband?" came her judging voice.

"Oh yes," JD said. He held my hand and looked glowingly at me. Her eyebrows were halfway to her hairline. And then I laughed. This appointment wasn't going well.

"Well, the father's date of birth then. . . ." she tried to continue.

"I don't know."

"His age?" I looked at JD. I thought Mandel was in his early forties. But I wasn't exactly sure.

"Listen," I said, halting the inquisition, "I just wanted to see Teresa and find out if she is the right person for me to work with."

"I see," she said, not even pausing in her routine. "I need a urine sample, and these forms will need to be completed before you can be a patient here." I didn't want to be a patient. I wasn't sick. I hadn't even decided if I wanted to invite Teresa into this process or not. Finally I got through to this nurse that I wasn't going to be a cog in her wheel, and with all the professionalism of a bad Sunday school teacher, she told me I could sit in an office and wait. The office door had some other physician's name on it. I was ready to bolt.

Then Teresa came in, calm, smiling, someone my same age. She had been a student of JD's, and there was a swift sharing of the story. She listened, engaged, drawn in. Her nonintrusive style, the opposite of the woman whose thumb we had just been under, was exactly what I was looking for in a midwife. She shared information, we talked about philosophy of birthing and options and choices. She suggested if I wanted her to work with me, to schedule an appointment near the end of May. We would begin then. She suggested several books I might find interesting.

I asked about the office. It was stodgy and male and didn't fit her personality. As a nurse midwife, she said she didn't have an office, but used whatever space was available. She didn't say, but I could see there was a clear hierarchy in the group, and she was at the bottom. She was working through the barriers of external power and attitude. They exist in every workplace, but seemed so out of place to me in a health care group dedicated to serving women. It was clear to me Teresa knew the problems; she saw the barriers, and was constructive in her approach. Infiltration. Change from within. I recognized a sister.

I bought two books recommended by Teresa, one on pregnancy and one about baby's first year, one for us and one for Mandel and Alycia. In addition to several books, we got a CD-ROM with information we devoured.

I was fascinated learning the process of fetal development and growth. The heart forms first as a long tube and ties itself into a kind of a knot that becomes the heart. The intestines grow out along the umbilical cord, and then reel themselves into the body when the cavity has grown big enough. I learned week by week what was happening, what was forming, checking a ruler for how long our little creation was. We called Alycia and Mandel weekly to report to them what was happening.

They had a book Alycia's sister had given them, and we followed along together.

In late April I began to look for Mother's Day cards for Alycia. She had shared with me many stories of how that day had been a raw, stinging time for her. One year earlier, she had told me of being at work, of the corsages of other women celebrating their motherhood. Her voice was bitter, understandably and painfully bitter. Her suffering had no day, yet their joy had this Hallmark holiday. Someone gave her flowers, a person who knew her infertility struggle. The friend thought helping her celebrate, even in the midst of infertility, would be a good thing, and it was, but thorny too. There was no way to erase or pretend or rationalize. There was no child in her arms. This year, I wanted to celebrate that though there was yet no child in her arms, there was a child. I found cards and sent her one from me and another one from the baby. I wanted so to affirm her connection to the life that was growing in me.

Mother's Day came, never a favorite holiday for me. Since my own mother mostly didn't like the day, I hadn't often celebrated it. Just a card for her with some honest appreciation was enough. While I was a pastor of a church, I felt the emotion loaded into that day and tried to walk with all people: the man whose mother just died, the woman whose children were lost to her, the ones who could not or did not have children, those whose mothers were abusive and destructive. And I also walked with the happy ones, those with lovely small children to bring them macaroni glued to construction paper, those children with arms that circled the neck and wet lips to push against cheeks. The pregnant moms were always shy but proud; the mothers with newborns haloed in light. "How many people here are great-grandmothers?" A few proud ones would stand. "How many grandmothers?" Always a new one startled that it was her turn now to change categories. "Mothers?" Many more would get to their feet, the veterans taking kids and books and stuff off their laps. "Now, anyone who ever had a mother." I would usually have to repeat it. The rest of the routine was well known in midwestern Protestantism. "Anyone who has ever had a mother please stand." And when everyone was up, we would say a prayer of thanks for the good in those women, for the joy and the pain of being children and parents, thanks for life itself and the mystery through which being alive comes to each of us.

Mother's Day was here—did I stand up this year if asked? Did I celebrate? Was I a mother? What I clearly thought would be a "no" in me wasn't so clear. I knew I wanted to celebrate Alycia as a mother-to-be, as this child's mother. And I knew I wanted to celebrate something new in me, a part of me barely forming. Along with the developing fetus, it seemed I was developing some new way of being me.

My sister, Laura Jean, sent me a wonderful card with a nesting bird and three blue eggs. She asked if I felt like a nest and gently said if I was celebrating Mother's Day, she thought this could be my card. My husband bought me the first dozen red roses I had ever received in my life. I felt proud as the day dawned: proud of my body's ability to conceive, proud of my courage to conceive this idea, proud of my risking myself for the sake of every-one's gain.

I watched the mail for word from Alycia. I listened for the phone. There was silence. A big silence. I was confused by this. Were we in this together? Why would she not be celebrating with me the same way I was want-ing to celebrate with her?

I don't understand infertility, but I do know what it means to be single and childless in a world of couples and families. I know feeling left out of the flow. I know the exasperation of believing I can do something and yet consistently failing at it. But I do not know the precise wound of infertility, this particular betrayal. Our sexual organs, our places of regeneration, are powerfully con-nected to the core of our souls. Infertility stirs deep places and agitates our self-confidence and our sense of self. They are not simple issues.

I had asked Alycia frequently in this process what she thought it would be like, and now what it was like for her to have her husband's child gestating in me. Was there instinctual jealousy? I would expect there would be. Was there anger at me for conceiving quickly and easily? She said no. Over and over she said no. That answer didn't make sense to me.

JD and I drove over to see Alycia and Mandel later in May. We had planned a visit back and forth each month and phone calls each week to keep contact among us. We drove down the long two-track driveway into their meadow of a yard. The house sat in a corner of the lot, looking like an old farmhouse.

We knocked and were told to come in. Alycia captured me with a joyous hug and cleared her tears and didn't let go until she sang a little Brazilian lullaby toward my belly with her head on my chest. I felt like an intruder in an intensely personal moment. Later I wondered about my reaction. What made it seem as if I was intruding, when six weeks earlier we had done what appeared more intimate without that feeling?

To celebrate the conception we went out to dinner at an Italian restaurant. We toasted each other with three raised glasses of wine and one raised cup of milk! When JD and I paid for the meal, we did so with joy. And yet it seemed odd for us to be paying, for us to be sponsoring the celebration. It seemed odd that we were the ones who had driven the seven hours again to make the time together possible. Was it just that we were more able to be flexible?

I found a small sculpture of four people standing in a circle with arms around each other. In the center there was space for a candle. I ordered one for us and one for Alycia and Mandel. It seemed such a lovely depiction of the way we were holding open a doorway for this new little soul to enter the earth. I would wait to light the candle until the baby was born.

A few weeks later, I met with Teresa for my first real appointment. I liked her again, and the ease of the first visit continued. She did an internal exam and felt my uterus might be a little too enlarged, a possible indicator of fibroids. Uterine fibroids are lumps of tissue of various sizes in the uterine wall. They are very common; one-quarter of women over thirty-five have them. They often enlarge with pregnancy and can cause problems.

Within minutes I was in another room having an unexpected ultrasound exam. The technician said, "Here's your ovary," as I watched a TV screen, transfixed with being able to see my insides! "The other ovary is here, looks fine." She found two larger fibroids and several smaller ones, and she measured them, while I watched, amazed at the machine and at seeing my own body this way. Then with just an adjustment of the transducer she said, "And here's Baby," and I saw a little lima bean on the screen. "Looks fine . . . and here," and she reached to flip a switch, "is Baby's heartbeat."

Washu washu washu washu washu. It was stunning. I heard a bird in fast flight. The sound was coming from inside me, and it wasn't me. I saw the lima bean, minding every bit of its own business, being . . . being.

It was like looking into a dark night sky full of stars, or seeing an intricate flower blossom open. Life was forming. I was a cup containing the primordial soup that was organizing itself in me. It was holy. And this wonder was happening inside my skin. Within me, within the heart of my body, inside my womb. I was not prepared, and so I was lusciously surprised with the amazing tangible confirmation of my baby's being and health.

In the heartbeat of sound the relationship formed. I had chosen and made this come to be, but also I had been chosen. I admired the lima bean's audacity to start out this way, to start from two cells and to create from that a self-support system, tapping into the existing environment and adapting and adjusting my temperature and chemistry and physical structures to be what it needed. I felt deep humility and was wholly honored to be the matrix. There was the Mystery, in me.

In these same minutes I was also having the news confirmed that all was not perfect: There were fibroids in me. Waves of embarrassment and shame moved over me like gusts of prairie wind. My uterus was lumpy! I wanted my hospitable uterus to be beautiful and smooth, soft and strong, not lumpy.

If the placenta was on or near a fibroid it might mean a greater risk for miscarriage. Fear eclipsed the shame. "Miscarriage" is a word I hate, as if the woman drops or fails to carry the embryo. I strongly believed I would have a good pregnancy and birth, yet I knew the statistics for miscarriage were high, higher for older moms, and even higher now. The additional risk from fibroids lasts throughout the pregnancy and includes a greater chance for premature birth.

I left the office sobered. I studied fibroids. I heard a few horror stories. In one story a woman had a fibroid as large as her baby. In another story, a woman needed a cesarian because her fibroid blocked her cervix. In yet another, a woman had a lump like a grapefruit that protruded on her wonderfully rounded belly.

But I wanted perfection. I deserved a perfect pregnancy, a perfectly round belly. After all, I was special doing this amazing thing. I was being selfless and giving. What sensational delusions we spin. There are no guarantees, not ever. Not for the very Christian, not for the ones who exercise every day, not for those who think only pure thoughts or who meditate three hours a day. We are all in life together. It is in us. That *is* the miracle.

I called Alycia and Mandel then to tell them about the checkup. I was fearful to say I had heard our baby's heartbeat. We had talked about having all four of us hear it for the first time. They were disappointed they hadn't been there for the experience but understood that I needed to agree to have the ultrasound done for my good and the good of the pregnancy. I explained about the fibroids as best I could, telling them the worst it could mean and assuring them that probably it wouldn't make any difference in the pregnancy at all.

I was the giver of news. I was the sharer of the meaning of that news. They reacted to what I said with words of understanding and acceptance. There was an odd power dynamic: I was wanting their support, and yet I was the one who was offering them the information and the interpretations and the assurances. I wanted to be supported too! But there was no offer, no words that came through the phone lines.

We were, I think, mutually awkward about it all. What was happening was bigger than our plans. Already the ideas we had were being adjusted and changed by the realities we didn't control. Already our experiences were becoming separate: I was having one experience, and Alycia was having quite another. There wasn't one pregnancy we could share, but we were each having our own experience, our own pregnancy. And the sharing was proving to be much more difficult than we had imagined.

I watch *Star Trek*. I have watched the original, the new ones, the reruns, the movies. I'm not fanatical, but

I am passionate about it. In it, there is a race of humanoid people called Trills. At maturity, they are able to be united with second, smaller life-forms, symbionts. They are made for this and strive and study to win the honor of being joined. A Trill without a symbiont exists, but the full and complete life for a Trill is to be chosen to be joined. The other life-form, the symbiont, goes into the Trill's body, and the two beings share the one body.

When the baby began to be real for me, I thought of myself as a Trill. I had two heartbeats! I didn't feel invaded, and I didn't feel as if I was creating another person, which are the two things I thought I would feel. I felt like another whole person had joined me, and for a time I would be plural. A Trill!

Although I long for intimacy, I am also an introvert, one whose energy comes from times of being alone. I was living in a more intimate way than ever before with another person, sharing my body, not just in sexual moments, but all day, every instant. I was feeling strong and very much myself. The intimacy did not take my soul energy. That intimacy without energy loss could happen at all was mysterious to me; that it was happening to me was a complex learning, a gift I am still opening.

I tried to sense the baby, its person, its personality, its spirit. At the time, we were all talking about how the baby was probably a boy. No one was too invested in this, but JD had said early on how Mandel would be such a great father for a boy because of his quiet gentleness and comfort in the world of nature. Alycia and I wanted a girl, yet warmed to this idea of a boy.

In my mind's basement, where the unbidden tangled things grow, I knew that letting go of a boy baby would be easier for me than letting go of a little girl, for ugly reasons. There it was. So, we talked about the baby and saw a "him." It is the only way I am aware that I tried to build distance and detachment into the process for me. Luckily it didn't work!

I didn't want to not love this baby, to hold back love for fear of the pain of separation. Several friends "remember" experiences from before they were born. Much is written on the effects of a pregnant woman's emotions on the developing fetus. Psychological or chemical, mystical or medical, somehow things were communicated, shared, between the two of us in this body of mine.

I wanted the baby to know my love—the support and care of me, its first mom. What effects would grow out of this unusual beginning were hard to imagine, but I wanted this child to begin in a sea of love—my love, my husband's love, our love for each other, and the very real love Alycia and Mandel each held for Baby.

I talked often to Baby those first months, and through the pregnancy, telling stories of the love through which it was invited to the mystery of life. I didn't feel a presence in any spiritual way until much later, but I did feel responsible to Baby, and glad and ready to be in this situation with him/her.

In June JD and I went to Seattle to get treatment for his prostate cancer. He was to have radioactive seeds implanted into his cancerous prostate gland on a Monday morning. While meeting with the oncologist on the Friday before, we asked him casually if my being pregnant was an issue, so sure it wouldn't be. JD was a physicist, he was very familiar with radiation safety. We had read a variety of opinions about how the low radioactivity that would be present around JD would have negligible impact on a fetus.

Indeed, the oncologist told us, even this low radioactivity was an issue. It wasn't very common, he said, for a man being treated for prostate cancer to have a pregnant wife. We laughed and told him about the surrogacy. He told us we would need to sleep in separate rooms and maintain a distance of six to eight feet from each other for at least two months. There could be brief intermittent contact, but the highest risk time in fetal development was matched exactly with the time of highest radiation. Contrary to our best intentions, the pregnancy and the Brachytherapy couldn't be colliding with greater conflict. We would definitely have to make significant changes in our lives.

The Gift of a Child

We were a couple who never spent more than an hour without some kind of touching. We sat close and walked holding hands. We snuggled before sleep every night. I felt a monstrous tearing inside of me. This wonderful dream of pregnancy was costing me physical closeness with my husband when he and I especially needed that comfort and security. I felt selfish. I hadn't been a caring wife to have chosen to follow my dream at the same time we were facing the cancer and its treatment.

JD and I talked, and I swallowed my fears and feelings of failing in order to deal with his cancer. The realities for him were different. His body held cancer, nearly in the same place mine was holding new life. In bed that night after he slid away in sleep, I lay eyes opened to new levels of complicating realities. What was happening? Where had the joy gone?

After spending the weekend with friends, we returned to the hospital and a hotel on Monday. The Brachytherapy was an outpatient procedure. JD chose to have a spinal block. He actually watched a TV screen as the hollow needles were inserted, and the seeds were set in place.

He came through the procedure in top form, and I went to see him in recovery while he waited for the spinal block to wear off. The nurses enforced the eight-foot perimeter with zeal. My husband and I needed to be close, to comfort and reassure ourselves after the procedure. I wanted to touch him and kiss him and hold his hand. I was told to sit in a chair across the room. I glimpsed the frustrations that were to build over the next few months. How could we be in this situation?

My emotions were tender and fragile from my pregnancy, and I was feeling the frightening reality of prostate cancer and the procedure that had just happened to JD. I was separated from him—not only by nurses who would soon be out of our lives, but by a commitment to the new life within me. To act out of my love for JD put the developing baby in danger of malformations and diminished brain cell development. To protect the baby meant staying away from my sweet husband lying now in a hospital bed, a little too happy from the medications that would soon wear off.

Feeling returned bit by bit to his legs. He had only discomfort from the procedure, and was ready to walk around and finish some tests in the hospital. After the tests, we went to lunch, then back to our hotel to rest, on separate beds, and flew home that night on a late flight. We changed seats on the plane so we would not be next to each other, and we made sure he wasn't next to anyone else who was pregnant.

Everything changed. We had to learn to walk farther apart than was natural, talk at a distance, sit and watch the TV news from different places. We made a joke:

Most people worry about practicing safe sex; we worry about safe snuggling. The laughter was a lifeboat to lie in during the storm of realities that had capsized our ship.

We found and ordered a garment designed for those who work around radiation. It looked like a diaper with Velcro closures around the sides. It wasn't exactly "lead underwear" but close. We ordered it the day we got home.

Emotions flowed. I felt guilty for not supporting JD, angry for not being free to hold him. I was hurting from the isolation and distance of not being held myself, missing the comfort of touching in the night. I was trying to support my husband's healing from the seed implantation and the trauma to his body and psyche. At the same time, I was dealing with my own feelings about his cancer and treatment, my fears of his death, and fears that the treatment, chosen for its ability to treat the cancer with less risk of side effects, would still damage him. Impotence and incontinence were the greatest risks, and neither one was something with which JD wanted to live. I was worried about the way the treatment would affect him physically and psychologically.

One night, still waiting for the lead underwear package to arrive, we slept on the living room floor head-to-head with our feet pointing away. We just needed to have some closeness. The "snuggle pants" as we named them arrived the next day. They were a gift, allowing us moments of protected closeness. But they became for me a symbol of the pain of conflicting realities. They were hot to wear all night, and I wore them because one other side effect of JD's procedure was difficult and frequent urination. He didn't need to deal with Velcro underwear in the middle of the night.

I was glad the seeds were in JD's prostate. They were our ally in the fight against his cancer. His radiation levels were of no danger to other adults, no danger, really, to me, but potentially serious danger to the little one taking form in the midst of it all. He said, on most days, he was still glad we were doing the pregnancy. We found our way through the tangled emotions and bizarre physical constraints. It was like being taught— hour by hour—that we were not good for each other, that closeness was a dangerous thing. We survived, but were changed.

The power of patterns, the deep unconscious communications of behavior, go beyond our thinking selves. We knew the imposed distances between us were temporary. We knew two good things were causing this set of problems. But we were being taught by our constant keeping of distance and coming together only with protection. Something sinister, not rational but real, was seeping into our selves and our relationship. JD was not safe for the baby. I was there for him, but only at a distance. I was choosing a little inch-long embryo over my relationship with him. And there seemed no better choices we could make.

Alycia and Mandel were to come visit us in June. I was looking forward to their being with us, hoping that they could surround us with their love in this hard time of cancer and pregnancy. Alycia and I had been strong support for each other over the years in times of need. I needed that support now. The time that fit all our schedules was Father's Day weekend. I was delighted! Mandel would be with his baby for their first Father's Day.

I was excited by that idea, a father and his baby. And instantly uncomfortable. As much as I knew Mandel to be the baby's father, I had a hard time thinking about it. I didn't pretend JD was the father, I just mostly thought of Baby as genetically mine, not a mix. To think of myself as "carrying Mandel's child" was peculiar. Mandel is a wonderful man, but to be having such intimacy with the husband of a friend was anomalous. To have mingled genes with someone I was not emotionally or romantically attracted to or involved with was culturally incongruous. It just felt uneasy.

When talking about this with one friend, she looked worried and frightened. Was I playing around with reality on a serious part of this whole adventure? Wasn't I dealing with the depth of it? She didn't share further apprehensions, but I suspected there were some. Whether I would hold on to the baby seemed everyone's biggest worry.

When I talked about not wanting to raise this child, about knowing it would hurt to let Baby go, and knowing I didn't have any idea how much, people often withdrew. They smiled as if they knew what I was talking about and I didn't, as if they knew that this would become a disaster. My friend didn't behave that way, but she withdrew some, and I did too. It is hard to share something this unusual, even with someone willing to try to understand. It seemed hard for many friends to offer me support since they would never make such a choice in their own lives.

Perhaps my friend was thinking, like many others seemed to be thinking, there is something wrong with a woman who can give away her own child. Something that goes against all it means to be a woman, a mother. A woman unintentionally pregnant might choose adoption, one among many painful options. But how could any woman in her right mind choose to become pregnant, knowing she would give her own child to another to raise? I hadn't anticipated being seen as callous.

I can see how unsettling it might be to hear this story. If some woman could let go of her baby, then might some of our assumptions of mother love be illusions? Perhaps our own mothers would also have been capable of such a thing when we were born. I was tugging at a thread that might unravel some of the social weaving that makes the world feel safe.

And it wasn't just the mother-love thread. Alycia, Mandel, JD, and I were tugging at the thread that connected sex to procreation. Many people are taught the purpose of sex is to make babies. We had conceived a child without sex. Using in vitro in a lab seems medical enough, acceptable especially because it helps a married couple conceive. But, if average people can do this at home, the relationship between sex and conception is called into question. Also, this was an extramarital pregnancy. Our anti-adultery instincts certainly get alerted by that. And for some, the religious concept of virgin birth would not necessarily seem so extraordinary anymore. The same techniques we used could produce children born of a virgin. All sorts of threads might be unraveling in the minds of people listening to this story. When a situation challenges entrenched thought patterns, people can become very uncomfortable.

A regular church attender hinted at a related concern. Did I wonder, she shyly proffered, if maybe God was behind the lack of a baby for Alycia and Mandel? Perhaps there was a reason for their infertility. If so, then was I running the risk of going against God, of somehow working against God's plan? This would put me in a bad situation, she suggested, one that would only bring me pain and suffering. I was touched by the genuine concern and the courage it took to raise those thoughts. But I have a very different view of God.

All I know of the Holy One leads me to believe that God is on the side of impossible odds, of dreams coming true, of the act of creation. God the prolific life giver, the great compassionate lover of all, the one who time and again pulls wiggling rabbits out of the hat of despair—I could not see this God being anything but pleased with our solution to Alycia and Mandel's childlessness. Besides, our experience was clearly that of being guided by this God who put stars to twinkle in even the darkest of nights, and who has promised, and delivers every single time, a sunrise at the end of each night.

A few days before the June visit, Alycia called and said they wouldn't be coming. She said Mandel wanted to be with his father on Father's Day. I said I thought he would want to celebrate his first Father's Day as a father himself, and be with his baby. Alycia understood me, she sounded as if she wanted to come, but said he wanted to stay home. I was torn but didn't want to interfere. My heart jammed with swirling images of my own father who was at best an absence, not a presence in my life. I found myself falling into the tumble of those feelings and old memories. I decided not to push Alycia. Obviously I had my own issues. I just accepted their need to be away and wondered what was underneath.

For them. For me.

I hung up the phone. I was beginning to experience another layer of myself. I saw from a new perspective. How could Mandel not be with this baby? was how it surfaced in the sea of my conscious-unconscious self. Underneath, I knew it had to do with my own father, his emotional absence and his painful neglect of me as a child. I did not dump the icy load of my conflicted childhood on Mandel's and Alycia's heads. I remembered it and released it all, one more time.

We took a trip to visit friends for the Fourth of July. The Beckers are in that magnificent circle, the ones who know how to truly love. Their home is a haven for the soul. JD and I drove seven hours across the plains, along blooming expanses of sweet clover, over the glittery water of reservoirs on the James and Missouri Rivers, along lonely expanses of lovely arching land. We came to our friends' place, and JD and I found support. They listened to us and laughed and joked with us. They hugged us. There was extended family there for the holiday: the daughter, her husband, their three girls who lived eighty miles away, and the family of their son who lived close by. The mother of the little girls said, "You have so much good on the way." She told me feeling the baby move was wonderful. Her daughters and I shared lighting fireworks. I helped the little girls to get in on the action and participate with the boys and men, not just let the guys do it. The wonderful men in this gathered family were more than ready to welcome the little girls. It was healing to be in the midst of that family.

Nothing was aberrant there: a woman pregnant with the child of her best friend's husband and a man who is radioactive and has cancer in a private place? Sure, come on in! Our friendship surpasses any expectation I have of family. I was proud to be there, pregnant. It was good to be loved.

5
The Second Trimester

The morning sickness was gone at the end of June. I felt strong, an embodiment of womanly power. Tired all the time, extremely tired some times, but also genuinely content. Even when tired I felt a kind of vitality. I loved being pregnant! The second trimester was a physical, bodily experience.

Someone turned up the volume on my nose. I began to smell things that I had never noticed before. I could smell the garbage long before any nonpregnant person could. I could also smell the faint fragrance of the passionflowers we had blooming in our living room. I shared these things with women who had been pregnant. They smiled with similar memories and told me their stories. I was being initiated.

I like to eat. I don't really feel passionate about the

need to eliminate all the fat from my body. I enjoy and revel in great tastes and textures. Popcorn. Flan. Wild mushroom bisque. But in the pregnancy, there was a new relationship with food. I decided my way through a day's menu. Could I get enough protein, enough calcium?

The baby refused fish, seafood of any kind. I simply couldn't get it into my mouth. I began to enjoy drinking milk, something I had never liked. I really didn't crave unusual foods. I needed to make myself eat. I actually asked Teresa how I might add calories to my diet when my weight wasn't going up fast enough. The one time in my life I figured I had license to be big, and I had to look for ways to gain weight.

I was taking better care of myself because another's well-being was dependent on my nutritional health. Why hadn't I always been this careful, this thoughtful, this aware? I promised myself to keep it up even after the baby was born.

JD has a wide circle of friendship: colleagues, close friends, others who know him well. We freely told the story of the pregnancy. Many people were wanting to celebrate this pregnancy with us. Ours is a party house. We like to gather good people, provide ample food, drink, and music, and watch the magic of celebration. So we planned a gathering. Alycia and Mandel's failed June trip turned into a July one, and so the party was planned when they would be with us. The invitation read: "Come and talk to four people who made a baby!"

Alycia and Mandel came for a quick weekend. Their work schedules made getting away difficult, and they were wisely saving their time off for after the baby's arrival. It was not a particularly close time. The magic of the conception weekend seemed to be all but gone. Distance grew between us like a strange untraveled land. Maybe it is a land that is uncrossable. The visit was friendly, but not intimate. Alycia and Mandel were excited to meet our friends, and at the party they were wrapped in the circle of support we had been enjoying.

Alycia and I went shopping for fabric. She wanted to do some sewing for me. We both sew, and I appreciated the offer of her time and talent. So I bought some fabric and a pattern we chose together. Having sewn for her sisters' pregnancies, Alycia was excited to offer this support. We had fun looking for just the right buttons and thinking about the shapes of the women in the pattern book. We laughed.

After we got home, the conversation was flowing between us. I asked if Alycia and Mandel wanted to read their baby a story or cuddle with it, as best we could manage. They didn't think so. I remember thinking that it was as if they didn't think the baby was real. I was curious, after all their excitement earlier, why they appeared to show little interest in the actual physical manifestation of our pregnancy.

The Gift of a Child

We talked about how the baby would be developing hearing soon, how they might like to tape their voices reading stories so he or she would hear their voices from the start. They liked the idea. But, it never happened.

We talked about the tests that come up as options at this point in pregnancy. The week was approaching that amniocentesis could be done—a procedure that extracted cells from the baby's amniotic fluid through the wall of the mother's abdomen. It would offer clues about the baby's health. Because I was an older mom, this was especially important to consider. The risk for chromosomal abnormalities was small, but real. It seemed a decision the baby's parents needed to make. I was eager to involve them. They didn't feel the test was necessary. Since the information it could give wouldn't mean any different actions on our parts, and since there was some risk to the pregnancy from the test itself, they decided not to do it. Making practical decisions was easier for them at this point than relating to the baby emotionally.

Soon after we scheduled the ultrasound. This time we would all be present to see the miracles and hear the heartbeat. There is a window of time that is optimal for doing the procedure, and when I told them the date the clinic suggested, they each had conflicts with it. I remember feeling that they didn't yet have this baby in the center of their lives as I did. How could they? They wanted me to reschedule it to fit their needs better. Teresa, my midwife, was puzzled about why we had to change it. We talked about what it must be like to try to be pregnant from hundreds of miles away.

We visited with our good friends Mary, Tate, and their daughter, Katrin, one day. They had attended several births, and if a home birth were possible for us, we wanted them to be there to help. Mary had asked if perhaps I would be interested in sharing this experience with Katrin, who was ten. We talked about it, wondering if Katrin might like to be a sister of sorts to this baby. Alycia and Mandel had a special tie with Katrin from staying with them at the time JD and I were married, so they were warm to the idea. That day, we asked Katrin if she would be interested in taking on this role. She seemed to be. We looked for ways of including her from then on.

August 3 came, the date for the ultrasound. Alycia and Mandel again made a quick trip over. JD and I picked up Katrin, and we all headed over to the clinic. What a curious and wonderful family group we made in the waiting room. Alycia and Katrin, Teresa and me all gathered around the scale as I weighed in. There must have been a trumpet sounding somewhere: It was one of the few times on the planet when women have gathered around a scale cheering for a big number.

JD and Mandel joined us, and we fitted ourselves

like puzzle pieces into the tiny ultrasound room, all looking toward the small monitor screen. Baby was very cooperative and we got wonderful pictures. A waxy hand moved. We saw the curve of a spine. Baby flipped over completely, and we told Katrin, who was a gymnast, there was definitely a family resemblance. We saw a heart. What beauty and intricacy! Those four tiny chambers all looked complete and were working perfectly together. The technician asked if we wanted to know Baby's gender, and I said it was Alycia and Mandel's choice. They wanted to know, and she said with a great deal of certainty she thought we had a girl!

Outside, we sat in the waiting room, waiting for Teresa to see the test results and then talk with us about them. Alycia had some tears as she looked at the little black-and-white photo. Across the room from her, I looked at my photo of the elegant hand, the tiny face, the being so complete yet not able to sustain itself. She was so fragile. And I looked at Alycia. She was in such a vulnerable position, one requiring great trust. Her face was naked. I felt an urge to protect Alycia. Just then Mandel's arm wrapped his strength around her. When she saw me looking at her, she smiled, her love and tears flowing.

Alycia seemed joyous; and yet I felt there was sadness in her as big as a house because these miracles weren't happening inside her body. Alycia seemed far away from me, even though the waiting area was small. I couldn't think how to cross the space in any new way. I think for her the pregnancy started to be a little more real in those moments. Dealing with emotional issues isn't always done gracefully.

The news from Teresa was all positive. The measurements were made to see if there was obvious signs of Down's syndrome, and that looked clear, too. A healthy baby! A healthy baby GIRL! Everyone warmed up to the new idea of a daughter quickly.

Next stop that day was at the records department of the hospital. We had arranged to sign the forms that would declare Mandel was the baby's father. Mandel, JD, and I each had a form. This assured Mandel would be listed as father on the baby's birth certificate. With his paternity established, the hospital would also be able to release the baby to Alycia and Mandel in the event of my death or if I needed an extended hospital stay. The forms were also some insurance that Alycia and Mandel could travel home with their baby without fear of someone challenging their legal right to do so.

Back home we were all standing in our kitchen talking about the ultrasound. Alycia's eyes were bright. Her face looked eager and open. Mandel's tall frame leaned against the counter, his curly greying hair and dark eyes, his smile as big as his heart. When I looked at him, I still felt shy. And yet I noticed him looking at me. And I imagined that with his quiet nature he was more shy than I was. And still, this loveliness inside of my body was his child. And I sensed that the little being was real to him now in new ways. Perhaps seeing the image—the tiny stubby fingers, the elegant face—and having watched her move made it easier to think that something was really happening inside my belly.

I wondered if Mandel would want to touch my belly. Alycia could easily do that. My relationship with Mandel wasn't that intimate. I shared these thoughts, and when Mandel indicated he did want to touch, I asked Alycia if she would help be the bridge again. Alycia took his hand and placed it on my tummy. He held it there a moment. My belly was rounded, and the solid roundness is always a surprise to someone who hasn't felt a pregnancy.

I felt a butterfly wing flutter, a fish tail flick. It was the first time I knew for sure Baby had moved inside of me. Mandel didn't feel it but he was right there, so was Alycia. His face looked like Christmas! He smiled wide and warm. Alycia's face filled with wonder. The first time I felt Baby move was when she was being nudged by her daddy's hand.

I was so glad that Alycia and Mandel were with me for that moment. I felt, too, a shadow to my joy. The frustration and waiting for a child had been endless for them. Now to be so close, to be inches away, and still not be able to feel what I could feel, not be able to touch this blessed child of their hearts, what exquisite pain and joy all mixed together. I wanted to share this with her, and so my frustration was real too.

We talked about how amazing it was to have had that moment together. No one would ever believe that it happened just like this, we thought. We each walked away feeling grateful to have shared that moment.

Sometimes the joy of being pregnant was overwhelming. I would sit quietly in the morning or walk in the yard feeling the deep privilege of being so near Mystery. Within me a being was forming herself! The biology is astounding, as is the psychology and the spirituality. I studied and learned what was happening and then in those quiet moments, I felt myself slip past being amazed and into awe. The whole Mystery was happening inside my body.

In August I went to see my friend in Maine. While there, I took my baby daughter on a whale watch. I had enjoyed seeing whales often when I lived in Maine; and so I wanted to have this little family outing (of sorts!) while I could. It was wonderful. I met several strong women on that day trip. I still had to tell people I was pregnant then, especially under sweaters and jackets, and they loved to hear our story.

I talked to Baby and told her we were on the ocean and would be seeing the huge beings called whales.

When the whales came it was wonderful. I felt good to be doing this silly thing. I knew Baby couldn't share the experience with me in many ways, but we did share everything. Emotions are chemicals, and much of our chemistry was shared. I stood on the boat and moved with the waves and felt the swells. There is something that happens out on the water that is primal and prenatal. Evolutionally, we emerged from that water. Taking her out on the ocean at that time in her life was right.

Being pregnant in the presence of the whales was great: their silky grey bodies surfacing for air, their sea-scented breath, the slapping waves and wind in my ears. There is such beauty in their rhythm of breathing and diving, of lolling near the surface. Such power in them exhaling, at three hundred miles an hour, two refrigerator-sized lungs full of air, and diving for the deep. The size of these animals infuses me with humility. Their quietness, their power, their enormity manifest as gentleness. I like that we are not so important to them as they are to us. I liked being near them, to introduce my little one to these tremendous beings.

I related to the baby as a separate person. And she was. I noticed that I was feeling like her mom, her first mom, and I was trying to do that relationship well. On the way back into shore, it began to occur to me that this new life would outlive me; that she would grow and live and be her own self. I wanted to know her; I wanted to see what life she made for herself. I wanted to bring her out on the ocean again, when she could stand for herself and see with her eyes, and tell me her own understanding of humpback whales.

All the eggs a woman has in her life are formed before she is born. Baby's eggs, the ones that would mark her month by month for the whole middle part of life, that might become children for her and grandchildren for me, they were all inside me now. It was a powerful idea, suddenly more than theoretical. I tried to comprehend. Nesting dolls, one fitting inside the next, suddenly made sense.

Not surprisingly, on the plane home, I thought of my own mother and our strange relationship. I knew this egg now growing as a baby was inside of her before I was born. I settled for that connection, one of tenderness in thought and remembrance. My mother and I were seldom in contact. The announcement letter I had sent out in late May went unacknowledged until September, when she sent four sentences in a card, one of them about my pregnancy: "Isn't it the best and the worst of times?" Something like that.

My mother and I had once been close. I gathered those other memories: the laughter and the talking, the smells of cinnamon bread, time sorting through wonderful fabrics, talking about ideas. I held those things close. This was a time I wished for a different reality with her, wished for there to be less distance and more laughter and cinnamon. But our paths were far apart. What I wished for was not in the real world. There was sadness for me, and the awareness of opportunity lost.

Other people told me they were proud of what I was doing. The words of support and understanding came, but often not from the places I expected. Not from my mother, not often from Alycia, not from her parents. But I did get the words and encouragement I needed. Many people wrote cards. A former parishioner I hadn't heard from in fifteen years who had adopted a daughter told me what a gift I was giving. A friend praised JD and me for "offering our lives for this great need."

But support wasn't often there as I wanted it from Alycia or, with the exception of my sister, from family in general. Several key friends were oddly silent. I do not know why. I have learned through other experiences to broaden the net when thinking about family and to accept the love that comes, no matter the direction it comes from. I was not without support or encouragement, or expressions of love. It did often come from unexpected places. I think that was a teaching about trust.

JD was great with me. He gave kisses to the baby when I wanted to but couldn't reach. He tolerated the snuggle pants I still wore to be close to him. He began wearing them himself as his symptoms from his cancer treatment eased and as my belly grew larger. With those as a barrier we could be close. He held me. I began to feel a dependence I never had before. A need for regular and repeated reassurance. A need for a secure home base. A need that he would be there for me. And he was.

One way I responded to my need for a secure home was to can fruits and vegetables that fall like a madwoman. Peaches, tomatoes, salsa, spaghetti sauce were just the beginning. The hard work was a tie with generations of women who canned out of necessity. I admire those tenacious women. The sound of the snapping lids as the jars cool, the sealing in of summer, brings me joy. I couldn't stop canning. Perhaps it was partly the nesting thing, being sure I had enough put up for later. Instincts are curious.

JD's birthday is September 13. He was sixty-five. We had a grand celebration. We sent out invitations for people to come and join us in marking the rite of passage. We said, "Remember how it felt when you were turning eighteen and the whole world was waiting for you on the other side of the doorway? Well, sixty-five is like that too." We roasted a pig, and I baked a fabulous 62-foot-long cake with sixty-five candles all in a row. We made salads and baked beans and invited our very favorite musicians to sing.

Seventy-five people were inside and outside the house. There was laughter, the joyful sound of people talking over common food. There was a spirit of admiration for JD that flowed among the gathered family and friends. I danced with some women and girls in the backyard when the music was irresistible and felt the baby dancing inside me.

JD, touched by the occasion and by the heartening presence of people he loved, gave a speech about living life fully. His cancer treatment was going well, and his life was being given back to him. He shared the learning, inspiring many younger ones to see the future as a time of continuing growth. People gathered in joy. It was a good day. We had leftover pork for many months. And I canned those extra baked beans as soup. But mostly, afterward, we had love stored up in our hearts for a long while.

The package I was waiting for finally arrived from Alycia, and I was eager to see the clothes she had made for me, expecting to be delighted by her considerable talent and her lovingly crafted gifts. Perhaps here would be the stitches that would sew our experiences together in this pregnancy.

Disappointment overwhelmed me. The items were wonderfully made, she had even finished the seams. But, she had changed some things. A piece of wool we agreed she would make into a jumper, a piece of fabric I had saved for years to be a jumper, was cut instead as a tank top. I didn't like that! It didn't even seem useful. The denim jumper had a flaw in the fabric right on the front shoulder. It seemed that could have been easily worked around. I tried on the two shirts whose fabric and buttons I had bought that day we went shopping together. They were several sizes too big, and just hung on me. With all that had been invested, there was only one usable item in that box.

I was angry. I was hurt by what I perceived as thoughtlessness that was causing problems between us. Still the clothes were there, gifts given. What a complicated reality in which to live.

I was planning to go to Alycia and Mandel's for a visit in September. I wanted to address some of these concerns and hoped maybe we could get back on the path on which we all wanted to be. I offered some possible dates, and they always had conflicts. Once, when we thought we had arranged a time, they canceled it. I was disturbed that they didn't make room in their schedules to see me.

When I shared things on the phone about my midwife appointments Alycia was appreciative, but she didn't often ask about the pregnancy or initiate the phone calls. My fears were growing as my visit to them got pushed back farther and farther. By the time we were trying to see if I could visit in mid-October, I decided to write Alycia to share what I was feeling. Phone calls had become difficult and distant, and I was so emotional

The Gift of a Child

I hoped that in a letter I could say things more clearly.

I sent the letter during the first days of October, and waited to hear. But I didn't. On the phone, when I asked, Mandel was angry because the letter had made Alycia feel bad and cry. Alycia said she was going to answer it, but wasn't ready yet. I decided to give up on a trip to see them. It seemed I was the only one trying to make the visit happen, and the dates under consideration were now in late October, when the weather was cold enough that there could be ice on the roads.

The perfect little group was like a lump of clay on a potter's wheel that was off center. I wondered, because I wasn't being told, just what was going on. Was their marriage in trouble? Were there some terrible fears at work? When I had assured them about my feelings about the baby, that I was loving her and not wanting to hold on to her, Alycia seemed to believe me. I had tried to be conscious of what I could do to be her friend in this time, but I wanted the same consideration from her. Still, I looked over every detail: Was I doing something wrong? We had talked earlier about sharing the time of birthing. Of Alycia and Mandel's coming to stay with us for a week so together we could move through the transition gently. I was rethinking that. What could we do to regain the circle, arms around each other, holding open the space for the birth of new life?

Earlier, we had agreed that breast-feeding for a while

would be good for the baby. Alycia had blurted out, "Then I get to burp her!" I had cringed. I heard that conversation echo in my mind. I imagined this little child being covertly fought over. I knew I wouldn't do that. The person inside my body was not a doll. She was a complete human being in a way I hadn't known she would be. My respect of her wouldn't let me make plans like that. Again I knew that Alycia's ideas and attitudes might have been mine before this pregnancy. But my reality was changing. Pregnancy, for each of us, was a distinctive passage. It became harder and harder to share. I could no longer imagine trying to live a week with them in the transition or tag teaming breast-feeding and burping.

JD and I took a wonderful trip to the Black Hills in late October. There was spectacular weather, clear cool air, an electric blue sky, quiet days at a place that in the summer is infested with too many tourists. Many more animals than usual were down where the roads go, groups of a dozen deer when usually we would see one, mountain sheep in a mass. We stayed in a modern log cabin, splurging to treat ourselves, poked around the slag piles of abandoned mines for interesting rocks, watched a deer walk through the trees near our cabin.

I saved my energy for a hike into the hills to the tall granitic Cathedral Spires. After a steep climb, nearly impossible while six months pregnant, I stood on a flat high meadow in the midst of towering rounded monoliths. The air was incensed with lodgepole pine. Sunlight angled through trees. The place was high and above and apart. The accomplishment itself was exhilarating to me.

Always while there, we spend time with the bison. A small bunch was grazing at a crossroads, and we sat with them for a while. A soft, huge sound turned our heads as two hundred bison came tearing over a rise, and poured down the slope toward us at a dead run. They slowed, crossed the road, and walked and trotted around us. We were thrilled. We each have loved the bison for many years and have spent time sitting on the car hood in their midst as they graze and chew and walk the prairie. To be near the power and might of those animals is a gift. They are secure and grounded in themselves. It rubs off.

Another day we spent time watching four huge male bison walk around a small pond. They settled on a place near the road, near us, and I went and sat on the ground too, and JD took my picture with them. The bison lay down behind me. I laughed and curled down against the prairie too. JD took another picture. The smell of the damp soil, the dried grasses and sages, the earthy smell of the stones brought comfort to my heart. I am a prairie woman, and lying in a herd of ruminating bison was a perfect place to be.

Then there was a piercing cry, and another, and we

looked up to see eagles. A pair with a young one. There were three of them, and three of us. They circled for twenty minutes, and the quiet was filled with strength and power. JD and I, talking softly, opened ourselves to the wonder of this place, receiving blessings from beings of great spirit.

Two other golden eagles led us out of the park the next day. At one point they tumbled over each other in the air, something I had never seen before. We moved out of the magic as we left the cathedral that the Black Hills are, and things were just what they were again. We didn't talk: Our needs for recognition and support had been met. We were renewed and restored.

Our spirituality is broad. JD and I both have roots deep in Christianity. We both have affinity with other expressions of the Creator, the animals and plants, the stars and the thunder. JD and I are tuned in to multiple levels of the Spirit. I call myself bi-spiritual. Maybe more than "bi."

We sat in his physics office one day with a friend looking at spectacular images from the Hubble Space Telescope on a computer screen. Our breath caught. We were bolted together into a tiny community. JD switched off the lights, and we were, the three of us, on a flight of wonder as image after image was before us. The beauty of the universe overwhelmed. Power. Immense size and enormous power. Most provocative was the feeling of connection, the familiarity of the universe.

We saw light that had exploded farther away and longer ago than we could accurately comprehend and recognized it, knew it as beautiful. There is something I hesitate to name, whose presence is all I need. On a prairie, in a physics office, sometimes even in a church —especially if it is a small one, and people are honest about their hardships, and they are perhaps singing— paying attention is all we need to do. The power that sustains and reconciles and makes new is there.

6

The Third Trimester

November brought the need to prepare for the coming birth. I knew how much I was looking forward to this big event, and how many variables there were.

A birth is a natural event, like a storm, and cannot be planned anymore than a prairie thunderstorm. It can be prepared for. I considered many options and read birth stories. I often watched a daily TV show that told about one birth each episode. I cried with the wonder and growled at the way so much intervention was used. It amazed me how in the dominant culture so many people take over a woman's journey. I learned to hate the chanting of "push push push" that always was commanded of a woman. Much was intrusive.

My dream birth was a water birth in the hot tub of our own home. It made the most sense to me. I love the water and feel so at home in it. There would be comfort and support for me, the laborer, and ease of transition from water to water for the baby. I wanted a peaceful environment, a quiet place, a private space for birthing.

I wanted to labor with all awareness, to notice and feel it, to be supported but not distracted by the others who would be present. I did not want to be shaved or sanitized or cut. I wanted our rhythm to determine the stages of labor, the timing of birth, not a hospital's policies or a practitioner's schedule.

More than anything I wanted to give the best birth to Baby: to respect her, to follow her lead, to assure all people treated her every moment with honor and courtesy. No one would be tearing her away from me the minute she was born to be measured and weighed just because they always do it that way. And I wanted the freedom to move when I wanted to move, to eat if I wanted to eat. I wanted to have our labor and birth be ours.

I knew there would need to be compromises.

In South Dakota, midwives are only newly included in the hospital scene. They aren't "allowed" to attend home births. We felt as if we needed to be extra responsible for this child, and my age was a risk factor. An unattended home birth seemed irresponsible. I did keep it as a private option in my own mind, and we had the essential tools assembled. Teresa was by now an integral part of my pregnancy, and I wanted her there. We developed a plan of staying home until the last possible moment, then being in the hospital just as long as was necessary. I don't see hospitals as evil, but neither do I see them as necessarily safer or the right place to be during and after a normal birth.

I talked with my sister, the nurse, during this process. We talked through all kinds of possibilities and complications. She works at a large, conservative hospital and found my ideas interesting. She had taken one book I was using, *Birthing from Within,* by Pam England and Rob Horowitz, and passed it around at work.

We talked with our friends Mary, Tate, and Katrin about attending our labor and birth, and helping us through this time. Katrin came with us to the Birth Educator sessions. We didn't join a group because of the unusual circumstances, but arranged for a few private sessions. The Educator talked with Katrin about preparing for the sounds and the sights of labor and delivery. I had definite preferences. I wanted to stay active during labor. I wanted a quiet room with as few attending as possible. I wanted no medical interventions unless we had tried all other ways of solving the problem. We demonstrated to Katrin some ways she might give support as I labored. I worked hard at remaining flexible, at not getting my expectations so set that something unexpected would be able to derail me.

Communication with Alycia hadn't improved; there

was still no response from my October letter. I felt so frustrated. I thought I was doing the best I could to get the problems between us resolved. I was being direct and clear about what was happening for me. I was asking Alycia and Mandel what was happening from their point of view. But the answers didn't come.

I knew I could have softened my approach. I could have made more of an effort to see things from their eyes. I could have offered to help them put words to what they were experiencing. I knew how. I had often done that sort of thing in my friendship with Alycia. It was a role that I often filled as a pastor. But, in this situation, when it was me who was carrying the child and me who would be required soon to release that child, I felt I needed to be the champion of my own needs. I couldn't see how to become the peacemaker between the two couples and still be sure my own needs were going to be met. And, I couldn't require myself to give up any more. I had reached the edge of my capacity for giving.

Once clear about that, I knew what I needed to do. I felt a great sadness that the relationships were broken, but they were. I wrote again in early November, saying I was getting clear about how I wanted birthing to go. I was afraid to tell them these decisions. I was about to take something unrepeatable and precious from them, and I knew it. I did so with deep sadness. I wrote that because of the tensions and the unresolved issues,

I didn't see how they were going to fit into the quiet, safe, comfortable environment I was working to create for the birthing. I needed to be focused and felt that the stressful conflicts between us would make the birth more difficult for me and maybe even for the baby. We didn't have a recent history of ease, of supportive talking, of shared understanding of birthing philosophy. As it was now, I didn't want them in the room.

In addition, I said I would like to have some time alone with the baby to say hello and good-bye, to finish my time as her mother. Just a day. I needed some time to experience inwardly that I was sharing her, that she was not being taken from me. Being certain that I was giving, not being taken from, would make the break clearer and cleaner. In the long run, those plans would be best not only for me, but maybe even for all of us. And this plan would, at least, contain the conflicts and tensions. The baby needed to be the focus. She was our common ground.

It was frightening to suggest these changes, to admit the depth of my feelings of disconnection and conflict with the parents of my/our child. But I felt, given their silences, it was the only way.

I initiated a phone call two weeks after they had the letter. They read what I had written, and didn't like it, but also heard what I was saying. They showed a remarkable acceptance of my needs. We awkwardly made new plans. They wanted to be in the hospital when she was born. We agreed to call them as soon as we left our house for the hospital. I was happy to compromise where I felt able. I was glad for them to meet Baby soon after she was born. I wanted them to have some of those early times of bonding with her. I wanted the baby to look into the eyes of her mother Alycia and learn that face. I wanted her daddy Mandel's voice to be the one who whispered her to sleep and calmed her cries. But I wanted this ending to be right for me as well. I asked for what I needed. There were many needs that required balancing. A third party intervention might have made this easier. But by feeling our way through, ungraceful as it was, the decisions were ours; the learning, the growing were ours as well.

I gathered a group of women around me in mid-November to share, not in a baby shower, but in a time of support and exploration of the mystery of birthing. We drew our images of birth. They shared thoughts and wide-ranging experiences from the births of their children—gentle births, difficult births, twins. Some loved the experience of being pregnant, and moving through the process of labor, and some had no idea why I would be interested in going through pregnancy and birthing and not, then, have the child.

We were mostly church dropouts, though not all of us. We all had been raised and nurtured in Christianity.

In the midst of the conversations, one woman's face shed its social veneer. Moved by the power of what we were gathered to do, she said, "This is holy." She opened the door to a room that has few words. Those of us witnessing her statement saw the tears that wet the edges of her eyes felt the weight of the silence that followed. It was holy. God was in this. This amazing journey was within God, inside of the Great Mystery. The amazing giving, the sharing of life, the offering of self for another's good, the piling up of grace upon grace of mystical experiences, these were named. This is holy.

And all of us, each one, came down this path to birth. This special circumstance made the holiness so clear. Undressed of a couple's feeling of accomplishment "our love made this baby"—it was perhaps clearer. Gestation is a holy path.

This was so clearly a gifted conception, and a blessed-by-God pregnancy. To a large extent what I believe made that true was Alycia's enormous sacrifice. Frederick Buechner, in *Wishful Thinking: A Theological ABC*, says: "To sacrifice something is to make it holy by giving it away for love." Alycia offered up her unfulfilled hope and dream of being a mother—what enormous courage that took. Offering one's best is perhaps a fun thing to do, but to offer your weakness is extremely difficult. Her willingness to let her brokenness hold life was a powerful refusal to be a victim. My courage and willingness to give were obvious to many. But Alycia's courage and what she was called on to sacrifice were enormous, private, and likely the more profound gifts.

The talk of holiness within the women's circle grew until it included more and more of us, leading naturally from the time of making birth art to a time of expressing ourselves in ritual. Mary officiated as we shared in a blessing circle. As each added a thin ribbon to a necklace pendant of a bear, she added a word of blessing for me. There were tears about the loss that was coming. It was a time of shouldering the knowledge of loss. There were words of admiration for choosing to make dreams come true and encouragement for my coming days and months and years. There was support, and respect, and love expressed. I gave each one a votive candle in a glass to be lit when the word reached them that my labor had begun. I liked knowing lights would be there, shining for us.

After that the spirit of the group shifted again, naturally. The mood lightened. The focus returned to the coming new birth, and the accomplishment of finding my way through this land-mined endeavor. We ate lunch together. The fullness of life was there with us, not just smiling faces. We laughed and enjoyed the treasures of womanhood. It was like no baby shower any one of us had ever attended!

Then I got a letter from Alycia. She asked if we

could get together and talk the birthing plan through again. It was a few days before Thanksgiving, she worked as a salesclerk, and the holiday season made getting time off for her now impossible. However, I wasn't comfortable driving on bad roads for seven hours and being so far away from home as the due date neared. She wanted to resolve the conflict and end this pregnancy in the spirit it had begun. A worthy desire we shared. I had been trying to get that resolution to happen for two months. Now that she was ready, the circumstances seemed to make it impossible. I called and we said those things to each other over the phone. She seemed to agree what she wanted was not now possible.

We did the best we could. I wished we could have done better. I wished for Baby to be born into the wonderful spirit of her conception. But, I'm told ballet dancers have ugly feet, and they sweat. What looks graceful and beautiful often is painful and messy as well. Love isn't romance, after all. The realities were not as easy to choreograph as we had hoped. The dance not quite as simple and elegant. But there was grace. There was grace granted all around.

Beauty and perfection are not the same thing. There is beauty in the desire of Alycia to want to grab the baby tight as she emerges from birth and hold on to her forever. There is beauty in the desire of Mandel to protect and defend his child. I knew in my heart no one wanted anything that was wrong. But our desires conflicted, our needs overlapped. We had found a path that meant everyone could have as much as possible of what they needed, but not all of what any of us wished for. We kept the plan we had worked out on the phone before Alycia's letter. As things were, there really didn't seem to be a better way.

My belly was finally big! I had been waiting for this time of fullness, and I got it. I was healthy. Tired and healthy. Baby's growth was good, and I loved the roundness of me, the heaviness of my breasts and the tremendous space I took up. I reveled in it. We took my picture sitting beside a huge pumpkin, naked and laughing.

I was up at least once a night. Often the moon shining through the skylight above our bed made a path I followed to the bathroom and back. Walking the moon path I felt like a queen. Leg cramps also came in the night, a searing knot of pain that wakens one instantly and completely. Increasing my calcium for a few days stopped them.

Thanksgiving was at our house. We gathered with relatives, JD's daughter and family, and my sister and her husband. JD and I made all the traditional favo-rite foods. We celebrated the abundance. Again I felt the instinct to cook and provide. Our table was full. The feelings of being in the midst of extended family brought a deep comfort and assurance of ongoing stability in our lives.

My midwife appointments came faster now, and every time things were fine. We talked about our birth plans, and about the stresses of the surrogacy. We listened to Baby's heartbeat. I felt ready. I was even hoping for an early birth, so Mandel and Alycia could have a Christmas baby, but I knew a first pregnancy was likely to go longer than shorter, and the due date was January 4.

Teresa suggested I ask my sister about our family history of giving birth. I learned that our mother's labors had all been short, six to seven hours, and that both of my sisters had had labors that followed the same pattern. That was wonderful news.

I read that three hundred thousand women are laboring at the same time around the planet. What a communal experience of power and pain and work. I would love laboring in that communion of women, but I would miss Alycia, the one woman who was supposed to be by my side.

Teresa suggested that I think about something to call Baby when she was born before Alycia and Mandel would officially name her. Not a name, exactly, but something to call her. That night JD and I thought about a name together. My last name before marriage had been Bernard, meaning "brave like a bear." I had always loved the meaning of that name. And JD had been given a name, as he was adopted into the Arikara Nation: He was Matkuska, White Bear. This would be our Bear Cub, the little spirit child who was coming through us into the world. Cubs were also born in the months of winter, the time of hibernation. They were fierce and strong. The name was right. She would have this first name, Bear Cub. I found a silver talisman that I had been given years before, of a big bear and a bear cub together. I kept it close.

Bear Cub turned one morning end over end. It felt like the insides of my tightly curved belly were being turned inside out. She moved frequently, and I loved the feeling, especially when her movement could be seen on my belly. She responded when JD tickled her feet. She moved to music. But this morning was much different. She flipped over and lay breach (head-up and bottom-down) for a few weeks. Just as I was starting to be nervous about it, there was another total body flip, and she righted herself.

One pregnancy book declared her development complete on December 13. The rest of the pregnancy, it said, just added fat for good measure. This information took root in me. I had completed it! I was joyous, and we took pictures to celebrate. Being successful was a great feeling. Bear Cub was turning the corner toward home. Moving around by now was awkward. Getting out of the water bed took some interesting maneuvers! But all was well. The conclusion seemed on its way.

We had a party in mid-December for a group of

musicians that comes together once a year. They put together a program of Christmas music—contemporary, original, and spirited. Because of their giving natures, we had made it tradition to give back, to create a party for them as they neared the end of their two-week season. They are longtime friends of JD's, and friends of mine. It was fun to "make party" as one might make love. To be lavish with those who give of their talent and spirit. Our house was full of celebrating. There was laughter, good food, and playful music.

A few people talked with me about the pregnancy. One woman, in her forties now, who had given a child in adoption as a late teen, said with tears, "You never forget them." Her clarity and compassion were for the time of good-bye that was on its way. I thanked her.

Another couple stood with me. They knew what I was doing. They shared the wonders and the horrors of it and didn't back away into the world of questions and small comments. They breathed with me. It was intimate beyond words. Life is about moments like that.

Christmas. For so many years it had meant that I helped with Sunday School pageants, preached sermons, visited those with Christmas blues. For so long I had lifted onto my shoulders the obligations of making Christmas happen for a church full of people. As any parent knows, making Christmas magic is a heavy burden.

The Gift of a Child

This year I had no congregation, no sermons to write. Instead I walked around feeling like an embodiment of the whole seasonal message. One of my classmates from seminary wrote of what a precisely perfect circumstance it is to walk up to a pulpit and read those advent and Christmas texts with a lovely round belly pushing out your vestments. Indeed. Even though I wasn't preaching, I smiled thinking of being largely pregnant at this time of year. The unusual circumstances of this pregnancy, no more God blessed than all other conceptions, but sharing the oddness at least of conceiving unusually, made me hear the story of Mary with different ears. She too held a child not destined to simply be her child. Her baby belonged also to others, to all others. I can imagine Mary rubbing her round belly too, and savoring each moment her child was just her child.

Beyond the obvious identifications with the Christmas story, there is the theme at Christmas of incarnation: the Holy One taking form, the word becoming flesh, the high and mysterious manifesting in a manger. To me, that means however we know that Great Spirit, our higher power, the universe's energy, Incarnation means It seeks us out, It comes to us. Many expressions of spirituality inside and outside the major religions seem to be focused on us trying to reach out to the Power. Techniques abound for getting ourselves transformed, quieted, perfected enough that we can perceive the light, cleaning out our ears so we can hear the song. One thing I love about the Christian way of speaking about the Mystery is that God comes to us. It is so simple, so ordinary, so obvious. And that truth was never clearer than when smelling the spicy scents, tasting the sweet fruits, listening to the simple majestic music of the season while being with child. This child had come to be with me. She had manifest in my manger, had taken on flesh right inside of my body. And that is how God works. Exactly like that.

All these deep and profound beliefs were lightened by remembering a cartoon on a favorite seminary professor's office door. The drawing was of the classic Nativity scene: star, stable, wise men with camels, shepherds with sheep. Inside, Mary and Joseph flanked the crisscrossed manger, everything just so. The caption: "It's a girl!" Such radical humor isn't funny to everyone. But it recaptured the surprise we've lost through familiarity.

People seem ready to do spiritual calisthenics to prove their ability to be quiet enough in meditation, or to be true enough in belief, or to be pure enough in eating only organic, never synthetic. But if the Christians have anything right, maybe it is that the Force, the white light, the wholeness, the Great Mystery is seeking us. That's the great Christmas surprise.

For me, unencumbered with the giving I was so used

to doing, freed of the necessity of making it happen, perhaps I had the best Christmas ever. I allowed myself to be found more fully than ever by the only One that matters. Just breathing in the Christmas light, just having a cookie or two, just listening to some people make music that lifts them off the stage a bit, Christmas happened. My heart was at least as full as my womb.

New Year's didn't seem to have much sway. At a New Year's party I heard the same tiresome comments over and over, and felt awkward. I didn't know the people well. I put on a confident face and walked around big and proud. There had been a local TV news story, wonderfully done by Jayne Andrews, a sensitive and trustworthy reporter. The story made me a topic of casual conversation at the party. I told the story over and over. But there was little sharing. I got tired, and we came home. There was deep snow and we had some trouble on the roads, even in town.

A day or so later, Tate and Katrin came over. Katrin wanted to read her favorite story to the baby, and we had a good time together talking about her, and talking to her. Baby was moving enough that Katrin and her dad felt that marvelous evidence of a person within another person.

As January 4, the due date, approached I was eager to beat the odds and deliver on that date. A full moon, a storm system with a low pressure moving through—it seemed a perfect time for labor. I went out that morning to shovel some snow to see if exercise might get labor moving. There was a moderate amount of new snow on the ground.

I was just getting started, enjoying the feeling of working out in the clear cold air, when from two sides the neighbors' snow blowers converged on our yard. Their drivers never made eye contact with me. They cleared our driveway and the sidewalks. I just stood there amazed. I waved and thanked them as they roared off home. Those guys didn't know I was wanting to shovel the snow myself. I felt the recipient of true chivalry in its best and worst right then. JD was in the house doing dishes and we had a good laugh over the whole scene.

Late that afternoon I was all troubled. It wasn't going to be the day. I decided to go into the hot tub as I often did, just to be comforted by the water and to let it ease the weight of my uterus on the nerves Baby had taken to bouncing on from time to time. In that tub I gave in to the timing. I did some surrendering to the wisdom of the process. And I asked whatever listens to us in those moments, my wordless questions: Was Bear Cub all right? Would we do this birthing thing soon, was it going to be OK?

A picture emerged in my head, a presence strong and clear: A woman with a long wrap blanket coat, long messy whitish grey curly hair, eyes opening deep, and a soft smile. She was there. She didn't speak, but I heard her comforting, her assurance, her promise that all was and would be well. I relaxed, and received her message.

Then I asked in my mind, who are you? And I knew the answer as soon as I had asked it: a guiding spirit for the baby, to be sure, but she was also, she said, the baby's granddaughter. I don't know from where such pictures and words come. I'm not claiming magical powers or extraordinary visitation. I do know something in me or beyond me—it matters little which—was able to bring calm, to comfort my fears, and to connect me to a generational awareness that helped me take my place inside the Mystery.

7

A Birth in Three Movements: Allegro, Soli Dolce, Vivace Fugue Forte

Sunday evening when some Braxton Hicks (practice labor) contractions got regular, I thought we were on the way. I felt strong and wonderful. My belly would draw up tight and be hard as an inflated basketball. Walking made the contractions even stronger. I walked around and around the house, walked up the stairs and down the stairs, delighted that the time might have come. I stopped a moment in the middle of all the walking and wrote: There are butterflies in my heart.

This first burst of labor lasted several hours but didn't progress, eventually I had to admit we were only in rehearsal. JD and I talked to Teresa. The contractions faded, and I was feeling foolish for my excitement. Teresa helped me see there was nothing to be embarrassed about, some early work was getting itself out of the way. She praised me for my work. We all slept well that night.

The second burst of false labor lasted just a short time. It came the next night, and was something for which I didn't even wake JD. I spent the time wonderfully alone, had a cup of tea, and enjoyed my rhythms in the dark. The pain was such good pain—strong, clear, and confident. I trusted my body. I listened to what it was doing and knew somehow in my body there was wisdom for this. I would be able to do this amazing thing that was almost upon us. I rocked in my chair, surprised and completely sure that birthing was somehow in my body's canon of knowledge. I could trust myself.

I also felt anguish that night because, in order for me to have reached this crest of confidence and self-trust, I had needed to walk away from my friend Alycia, needed to leave her in the struggles and tangles that were keeping her from communicating clearly with me. She was not walking with me through my journey. I couldn't help her work through whatever was happening for her and still have enough focus and energy to be fully available for myself and my own challenges. There wasn't enough of me for that. I chose, I had to choose, to be there for myself, to fully run my own race, to not hold myself back in order to help my friend come along with me. I was already giving so much. I decided, against all societal norms, that I would put myself first. My confidence and self-trust emanated from that decision—if I was fully present for myself, I could do this! The unsolved distance between me and Alycia came from that same decision.

At my Tuesday appointment, Teresa said I had dilated two centimeters from the work over the weekend and the baby was down nicely against my cervix—all good signs that labor would be soon. She sensed my being really ready. She suggested some herbs that might bring on a labor that was imminent. I decided that to force Bear Cub to dance to my tune wasn't right. I could let her choose when to be born for herself.

I had wanted to encourage the labor in part because Mary, Tate, and Katrin planned to leave for a vacation on January 6 on an early flight. By Tuesday evening we were clear that because of the timing, they would not be likely to share in Bear Cub's birth. JD and I drove over to see them, and reluctantly we gave up the idea, promising to post things on our website so they would know right away. We wished them a good trip, and drove home.

I went to sleep on Tuesday evening around eleven o'clock. At one o'clock I woke, thinking in my foggy brain that my period was starting, which immediately woke me up. I got out of bed and went to the kitchen, where I could see a clock and have some tea. The contractions that greeted me were different. The disparity was like that between a store-bought tomato and a garden-grown one. These contractions were rich and full of zest! The sensation was entirely different. These hurt! I was excited. I found the rhythm to be every five minutes, for a length of about thirty-five to forty seconds. I savored the knowing for a while. This really was the moment! When the next contraction passed, I went to wake JD. We would have just two hours of sleep that night.

JD woke with a start, and was immediately supportive. He helped count and time contractions, and kept a record of the contractions so we could see the progression. We called Teresa to alert her. The hours moved by quickly. I breathed through the contractions, and JD breathed with me. In between, I rocked in the chair I was nursed in as a baby. I was surprised at how life was just normal between the contractions.

Being in labor was like being in love. I was in it. Labor was so vast that it contained me, it held me, it was my whole context.

I went to the hot tub, astonished at how much easier laboring was there. Relaxing into the contractions, or the "expansions" as *Birthing from Within* called them, was so much more possible in the warm water. To help and not resist what my body was doing, to work with the pain and release the tension—the words I had been reading for months made sense now. Even with the knowledge, it was difficult to stay on top of the pain, and not to surrender to it. Who was the horse and who the rider? It matters.

It seemed impossible to believe that a place that is usually one shape can become a whole different shape. My cervix was a tightly closed knot changing into a wide-open passageway. Not resisting the transformation was difficult physically, psychologically, and spiritually. For Western minds it is hard to feel that our rational minds are not in charge. Labor is an immersion into wisdom that is far beyond the limits of rational thought, or of psychological understanding, or of spiritual practice.

Soon I was having trouble keeping up with the contractions. It was taking most of the time between contracting to release my tension and relax and prepare for the next one. I entered into a perpetual state of concentration. Decisions were beyond me. JD and Teresa talked by phone. She came over and checked my progress. I was well on the way. After another hour or so, three contractions came right together, ninety seconds each, and we decided it was time to get to the hospital.

Moving out of the tub, I found the contractions much more painful. I was unnerved by the change. It seemed unnatural to be moving around, to be leaving the warm water. I needed help getting dried off and dressed. Over my complaints JD jotted a quick note on the web page, and we were off to the hospital. We arrived around six A.M., just as Tate, Mary, and Katrin were flying off on vacation.

Even though I had done all the preregistering, getting processed by the hospital was a tangle. Clerks were asking me questions I had already answered and didn't now care about. I finally said, "My contractions are a minute and a half apart and I need to go to a labor room now." They understood that. I wanted to be working and focused, not interrupted. Teresa was in the room when I arrived. I had a hard time getting comfortable or feeling oriented. We realized we hadn't called Alycia and Mandel in the flurry of getting to the hospital. I needed them to know what was happening. In the privacy of our home I was happy to let them sleep, but now that we were in the hospital, I needed them to know. JD couldn't make the hospital phone system work. We all had fluttery nerves! Teresa volunteered to make the call while JD went to move the car.

Just before 7:00 A.M. I started getting the urge to push. That's how they describe it, as an urge, but it is much more. It is as powerful as the contracting is. It is not resistible. I could cooperate, making it stronger, but my body was going to push.

I wanted to birth in a squat, a natural position for me. Surprisingly, I found that even having my knees bent up was totally wrong for me in labor. Something wasn't right about the arrangement of bones and spaces that way. I lay down on the bed, sad that I couldn't do what I had planned. I lay down because it was the easiest thing to do. Inside I knew I wanted to be low, grounded, on the floor not up on a bed. But to make that wish known now seemed beyond my ability. The experience had a profound and certain wisdom all its own. The thoughts I had just drifted through the events like smoke through trees.

Lea, a nurse who joined JD and Teresa and me, said to push, push, push, as they had told the women on TV. In the foggy place it took several contractions before I could tell her not to tell me to push. Her words were actually stopping my contractions. I finally did tell her; I even tried to be polite about it. Communicating with anyone took enormous effort.

Teresa asked my permission to break my water to see if it was all clear. I knew it was to check to see if the baby had pooped in the water, which might mean other medical people would need to be alerted. I agreed. The water was clear, thankfully. I asked to smell the amniotic fluid, and she got one of the towels and held it up to my face. A sweet, soft smell, an amazingly gentle smell flooded me with love.

The length of time between the pushing contractions surprised me. I could breathe and be aware in between, but in a blurry way.

Teresa said we were getting close to having the baby.

I suddenly, then, lost my feeling of being able to do it. It was as if I didn't know how anymore. I was the horse and not the rider, losing the advantage of intention. I had no time to think about why I lost my confidence, or what to do about it.

All of me was needed elsewhere. I suddenly wasn't present to the birthing but was caught in a nonverbal swirl of familiar painful emotion. I felt like I had been defeated, like I was stuck and helpless. The eddy of these feelings possessed me for many minutes. I grew passive. But, my body also wanted and demanded my attention: This was the birth! I was frustrated, but couldn't get my emotional feet underneath me.

JD gave me an image, "It's like white-water rafting," he said. "Make the most of each wave. Dig in and ride them for everything they are worth." That was the image I needed. I dug back into the labor and paddled through the racking pain.

A few contractions later, Teresa had me touch myself, and I felt the bulging head pushing my soft places out, an astonishing feeling. She gently said, "I think we are going to have this baby on the next contraction." And I decided I wasn't going to have another contraction. And so I pushed, slowly, and felt the burning pain of her emergence. "Slowly," Teresa said, and then, "OK"; and I felt every inch of her sliding slowly through me out into the world. There were sounds of spirit and joy from the five of us. Teresa lifted Bear Cub onto my lap. I could barely see because I didn't have my glasses on, but there she was.

She looked huge. She looked perfect. She looked as I had imagined her face to look. She squinted and cried a halting, choppy cry. We covered her and dried her a little with a blanket. Lea turned her on her side a little more as she opened her lungs to the air. We all heard those sounds never heard just this way before, the sounds of wavering announcement. "Oh, oh, oh" is all I remember saying. JD grabbed his video camera and captured those first moments.

Once she was dried, they clamped her cord. Teresa asked if JD wanted to cut the cord, and I said, "No! I want to do it!" I wanted the separation to be something I did so I would never feel she had been taken from me by someone else. Teresa guided my hand, and I cut through the connection, the physical connection, that tough, twisting bundle of veins and skin. "You're free! You're free!" The moment of birthing was complete.

They boosted Bear Cub up where I could see her better and sucked a little fluid from her mouth. We saw her quickly pink up. I smelled her. I kissed her head. I held her, wrapping my spirit around her. I loved her in a way I have never loved before. For many minutes we stayed like that, warm and calm and close. The nurse made her first Apgar scores (a quick measure of a newborn's health), while Bear Cub was snuggled against me, and later took her briefly to check and measure and weigh, but in minutes she was back on my skin.

I told Bear Cub that her heart was closing up the place it had used before to get her oxygen. It was learning to get her oxygen from her own lungs now. She had been through a hard time; I told her that it was mostly over now. She was safe. This new place was just the outside of where she had been, even though she felt she was in a whole different place. I hugged her securely and she snuffled and cried and learned to breathe. "Hello, little one . . . hello little Bear Cub." I slid my hand around that foot I had felt through so many layers just a day ago. Her tiny foot fit right into my hand, and she pushed against it. We breathed.

JD picked her up when we needed to deliver the placenta. He held her up to the window and introduced her to the world. It was a softly tinted winter morning that greeted her in the name of all that is.

Once it was delivered, I asked to see the placenta. Teresa showed me the home Bear Cub had made for herself, a beautiful translucent bag. Attached to it was a large, nearly dinner plate-sized disk that looked like a blood clot, rich and red. It was fascinating, but so alien. When did we lose touch with these normal parts of life?

Bear Cub was back in my arms. Nurse Lea took

some pictures of the three of us, then Lea and Teresa left the room, and it was just us in the warm, low light. We cooed, we rested. We talked softly. JD hadn't watched her come out of me, he said when I asked him what it looked like. He was paying attention to me. His head was right next to mine, I know.

We talked a bit more. Just phrases. We looked at her and watched her move. Slowly, very slowly, the world came back into our awareness. We called a few people. Bear Cub tried nursing a little. Her eyes were wide and true. She made little sounds. I love her. I told her that her mommy and daddy were on their way, that they were waiting for her and would be so happy to see her.

Bear Cub weighed seven pounds and two ounces. She was nineteen inches long. But she was so much more than those things. She was the fulfillment of many lives, the promise of many more. She was perfect. She was strong. Bear Cub's spirit was an old one, full of wisdom and depth and joy. And now we saw her hands, the fingernails we knew had been forming so long before. We saw the shape of her shoulder and her eyelashes and the soft abundance of hair.

I decided to get up and try the bathroom. Nothing prepared me for the surprise of feeling my internal landscape rearrange itself. It was another previously unimaginable thing. One takes one's body somewhat for granted at forty-two, nothing much new in the way of sensation. But to actually feel organs slide around against each other was fascinating. Those spaces recently full and round were ready to return to some semblance of normalcy, just like that.

A nurse came to clean up Bear Cub. We had a few visitors. I introduced this new little life to them and laid her in the arms of each one. The pediatrician came and examined her. She passed every test. Bear Cub and I never left that room. JD went home to put pictures on the web, to clean up, to change clothes. She was born at 8:19 A.M.; we were ready to leave the hospital soon after noon; and by 3:00 P.M. all the forms had been signed. We bundled Bear Cub into her car seat for the trip to the car. Into the room burst Alycia and Mandel.

I unbundled her and handed her to her mom and dad. There wasn't much ceremony. More cooing, more tears. JD took video. The five of us were wanting to regroup at our house as soon as possible for more time together. JD and I took Bear Cub with us, and Alycia and Mandel weren't far behind. We went home.

8

Saying Hello,
Saying Goodbye

I carried Bear Cub into our house. Crossing the threshold was powerful. I held her there where I had labored, where we had labored. We found her things I had collected—the few clothes, the diapers, the little basket she would sleep in. But soon there were people. My sister came. Alycia and Mandel came. Our favorite TV news reporter, Jayne Andrews, came as arranged to do a story for the evening news.

In the interview Alycia, who was choked with emotion, said, "I have wanted to be a mother for so long."

There was a pause; then I turned to her. "Ta da!" I sang. The magic had happened. Our whole journey was successful. She was a mother. She had a child.

We had a birthday party. The women from my support circle brought their families, came with cake and ice cream and a supper. My sister and I disappeared into a quiet place, and she helped us nurse for a while. We got better and better at it, and when we emerged, there was a whole quiet, loving party going on. Everyone saw the new little one. Alycia announced her name, Mylah Darrelle Johnson, and we sang the happy birthday song. I put a little drop of melted ice cream on her lips.

Although everything was compressed into a short time, profound things were happening one after another. One of JD's grandchildren kissed the top of Mylah's head with an unpretentious reverence that belongs only to children. A young girl I knew, the granddaughter of a friend, asked to hold Mylah. This almost teenaged girl held the newborn in her young arms. Her own baby sister had died in infancy a few years earlier. For those of us who knew the girl's story, the moment was especially poignant.

There were some gifts. One friend brought Mylah frankincense and myrrh in a gold and wooden box. It was January 6, Epiphany, the day Christians celebrate the three kings bringing gifts to baby Jesus. What a day for Mylah to have chosen to come into our lives. The gift of her, of life itself, the many gifts of motherhood and fatherhood, of birth, of memories and of hopes now began. She was a unique gift—for me, for JD, for her parents. Alycia and Mandel held her. They showed her off. They smiled.

I felt joyful to see her in their arms. This was what I had dreamed would happen, years before. They had a child. It was right. We were right: The four of us could make a baby. We had accomplished the amazing task we took on. Satisfaction is a funny emotion. There is a bit of "I told you so" in it.

Then around 7:00 P.M. everyone left, and we had another time of nursing. We ate the supper that had been given to us. My sister stayed with us overnight, and so we passed the little Bear Cub around between the three of us, reveling in her magnificence. I was up nearly all night, not wanting to miss any moment of Mylah's precious time with me. She nursed well, and pooped well. She cried some, and slept beautifully.

I slept a half hour at one point, and an hour and a half one other stretch, laying her in a little basket just a foot from my bed. She made little sounds, and I woke and heard each one. I heard her say she was ready for another time of nursing, and I gladly was awake and ready to respond. I only had this one day. Morning came. Faster than we knew.

Alycia and Mandel were to come to get her at 9:00 A.M. So after feeding her around seven o'clock in bed with JD, he took some wonderful pictures: her feet, her hand curled around my finger, her eyes looking up while nursing. He held her, and I photographed them together. He held her heart-to-heart. The tiny baby-ness of her was sweet, but the essential thing was her spirit, full and rich and complete. She was a sister to us, in that way. We had all lived together. Now she was moving on. The parting was taking up our focus. It was time for that.

First, I took some alone time with her. I changed her diaper, and marveled at her wonderful body. The softness of her skin, the shape of her shoulder; her toes were my delight! I held off dressing her, and tucked her inside my white terry cloth robe so we could be skin to skin and still stay warm. She looked into my eyes, and I promised her I would love her always. I promised her that even though she was living far away, we would still have a connection. Unlike the umbilical cord I had cut to free her, this other cord of connection would never be cut. I had tears, and I smiled. "I love you so, Bear Cub. I will be loving you always."

I listened to her. I opened to the communication of her. I didn't pretend to hear words or promises from her. I did feel her spectacular presence, the magnificence of her soul. We are all free and whole and belong first and perfectly to ourselves. I held that truth in my arms. She was a whole and complete human being, and belonged, in essence, only to herself. If anything she was my teacher that moment, and her "words" were those of greater depth and wisdom. Everything possible there was to say had been said. All the gifts had been given and received. The time for parting had come.

My sister came in and we dressed Baby Mylah. We cut a little of her long, soft hair, from the back where it wouldn't be too noticeable, so I could have something later to touch. I put her diaper in the garbage. Everything was wet with tears. That I would need to dump the garbage soon made me cry. Her diapers no longer with us. I managed to laugh at the inflated emotions, and dressed as my sister had some time with Mylah.

We gathered Bear Cub's things. We waited. Alycia and Mandel were late. I couldn't believe it. We gathered ourselves up to prepare for the agonizing moment. Then we had to wait. From my perspective that seemed too much to ask.

Alycia and Mandel arrived all smiles. They engaged in small talk, complained about their lack of sleep the night before, the night we were in labor, because their dog had been barking. They didn't ask us one question about the labor or birth. They didn't ask when she had nursed or how she was doing. They came in and just took a time holding Mylah and cooing at her. There was no apparent compassion from them for us, no acknowledgment of our twisting hearts—none that I could see or feel or hear. They were drunk on their joy. Who would have taken that from them?

We showed them the gifts Mylah had received. They

stayed. They chatted. I was dying inside moment by moment. I needed to get on with it. They needed to get up to the hospital to talk with the nurses about baby care. They didn't have any formula for her. I gave her the sample the hospital had given us.

Alycia said maybe I could just nurse Mylah again. I wanted to scream at the insensitivity. We were trying to say good-bye. I couldn't "just" nurse again in these circumstances, especially as a favor to her. Was I just a machine to them? Something that made a baby and now, in a handy way, could make milk too? "No," I said. "It is your time now to be Mylah's mother." I smiled, I think.

Finally Alycia and Mandel got their coats. It had been two hours. At one time we were thinking of doing this for a week! They bundled Mylah up and put her in her car seat. She began to cry. Everyone else in the room faded into pastels. I was frozen, leaning against the wall across the room, and Mylah was all covered up and crying, and no one was responding to her. They were talking about road conditions and travel.

Mylah! I wanted to go and bend to her, talk with her, tell her what was happening. I wanted her parents to be focused on her, to be responding to her cries, to treat her with respect. I wanted to go to her. But I couldn't. If I moved, I wasn't sure I could live through the pain of letting her go. So I stayed leaning against the wall, next to my sister. Finally—it had likely been only moments—JD went to her and rocked her car seat, and talked to her.

Alycia gathered their things. Mandel spoke to Mylah in the sweet voice adults seem to universally use toward infants; he spoke to her with the intimacy of a daddy. He was taking his place. I had to let her go. Mandel floated a plush soft blanket over the whole car seat, and Bear Cub was gone. Still they chatted. They smiled and laughed, seemingly oblivious to our anguish. I tried to smile too. They went out the door. It closed.

The moment was first silent. Then each of us—JD, Laura Jean, and I—all made the throaty animal sounds of pain; we huddled together, we sobbed, we comforted each other, we said what we needed to say. The car doors slammed. The motor started. We had more tears, more words of good-bye to our dear little one. Something stretched and stretched until it could stretch no more. It broke, and she was gone.

We didn't rush the tears, didn't indulge them either. We had some tea. It was quiet. We talked and didn't talk. Together, we passed the day. I don't remember much. They say you forget the pain of birthing, but it was this pain that has mercifully blurred for me. There was nothing to feel; it was the nothingness that was there to experience. The absence. Her little body was with me a day, but her spirit had been with me a long time. The house was unbalanced now, without her gigantic wings.

I was physically feeling good. What an advantage that was. It was Thursday, January 7. We tried to remember things like the date to find a way back to the world. We watched television. We tried to talk. The three of us were kind with one another. Flowers came—wondrous roses edged in pink with a pleasant note from Laura Jean's husband. There were flowers from JD's daughter too, and there was a plant from the attorney we had gone to see.

It felt like a house after a death—the vibrating air, the slow disorientation. We had to keep remembering Bear Cub wasn't dead. Our story ended with success and with joy. This pain wasn't exactly grief, but it was something close. What was lost was so much less than what was still alive. She was alive, our Bear Cub. Our Mylah. She was going to her home where she was supposed to be.

Alycia and Mandel drove back to Wisconsin the day they left our house. The roads were partly snow covered and had ice patches on them. It was very cold. Car trouble might have meant disaster for an infant just beginning to learn to regulate her body temperature. We didn't know exactly when they would leave town, but wondered if we might hear that they had arrived home safely. We didn't. We wondered if the next day they might call. They didn't.

strong, has space in it. Space for each one to grow. Our love is strong and can hold this big space of separation.

Not even forty-eight hours ago, seconds after your birth, I cut the cord that tied us together. I held the scissors and cut through the strong, fibrous cord that carried blood and nutrients and oxygen back and forth between us. I cut through it and said, "You are free!" And I felt the launching of you into your next time of life. I felt the completion of our "tied time" and the beginning for you of a new life, the beginning for me of a new time too. I felt joy. I feel it now in the midst of the pain of missing you. You are launched, you are loosed, you are freed into this world to do your teaching and your learning, to do your loving and giving, to be your own self: side by side with the rest of us. You are our sister now, another whole self.

So on this new day, Bear Cub, grow stronger. Breathe deeply. Stretch your strong muscles. Enjoy your freedom. Explore your new time and place. And know I am here, that I remember what we have shared, that I love you with an open heart.

Mama Bear

The Gift of a Child

I went back to bed for a while. I woke to hardened breasts: My milk had come in. With it, a powerful desire to get in the car and go to Wisconsin and feed my baby. Those instincts are strong, powerful like the need to breathe. I knew I wouldn't go. I savored the pain as an evidence of love.

I thought that I would not feel like a mother after Mylah went home. That I would lose my sense of being a mother, but it stayed. What left was the immediacy of her, the tangibleness of relationship. But she left me changed, and I stayed that way. I thought I wouldn't. I thought those feelings of having a baby would be gone when the baby was gone. But, I had a daughter. She was home safely with her parents, and I had a daughter. It wasn't what I had anticipated or expected.

My sister went home. The leaving was hard. Before she left, we had a long talk about the labor and the birthing. I told her about the experience of knowing what to do through labor, until all of a sudden I didn't, and I was stuck. She responded, but I didn't hear what she said. I just heard what I had said. I was stuck, I said. *I* was.

In my birth, while my mother was lying there drugged as was the practice in those days, my birthing progressed until a point when the doctor decided I wasn't coming fast enough. He decided I was stuck. My head was grabbed by metal spoons. I was twisted and pulled on and dragged out into the world that blasted me in bright lights and loud sounds. I know because I have marks on my head in front and in back. I know because that is how things were done then. It was usual.

I was stuck when birthing Mylah in the exact same place that I had, as a baby, been defined as stuck and was then "rescued." I stopped my sister, apologized for not listening to her, and explained my thoughts. The coincidence made sense; I was stalled in my progression of giving birth because I hadn't experienced that part in its natural form before. In that instant, I had become myself the infant instead of the mother.

Because I birthed in the presence of caring and mindful adults, I was allowed to heal this old wound. I was not rescued from my fear, but was encouraged to work through the fear, to engage the untraveled passageway just inches long that led from the inside of me to the outside of me. I found that "stuck" could be "unstuck." I was allowed to physically triumph through the time of faltering, and I learned in a physical way what I had not known before: How to be born. How to get out. How to finish on my own power, not to wait for rescue. Because Teresa was wise and JD was loving, I healed a trauma without words. I could never have identified my old trauma except by going through childbirth and by reflecting on it in all honesty and courage.

Laura Jean listened. She heard me. She didn't comment. We are different. She is much more practical, not so given to wild synthesis of life's depths. She has a wisdom I do not. I respect our differences. So does she. Love is like that.

Later in the day my breasts hurt. The pain was unfamiliar, another unknown. Ice helped numb it. I decided not to express milk so the process would be over sooner. I tied a dishcloth around my chest and asked JD to tighten it as hard as he could, and that helped some.

On Friday I panicked. I needed to have something of Mylah to see, something to touch. We had taken all digital photographs. I felt as if there were no baby, and so there needed at least to be pictures. We looked through all our photographs on the computer, and printed images—her feet, her face, her hand, her whole naked self, me holding her minutes after her birth. We put the pictures around the house. That was some comfort. The pink knitted booties she had worn held her fragrance, and I breathed as deeply as I could, like taking in a drug that would take away the hurt. I fought the urge to drive to Wisconsin. I cried.

Friday evening Teresa called and asked if she could stop by and visit. She asked if Alycia, Mandel, and Mylah made it back to Wisconsin OK, and I said I didn't know. She looked at the pictures. We cried. She gave me some gifts. We talked through the birthing time, how well it had gone, how it wasn't perfect but it was perfect too. And how beautiful Mylah was and how strong. Her Apgar scores had been great, a good healthy start.

We talked about how I got stuck in the labor, and what my new understanding of that was. Teresa confirmed that stories like that were common. Her smile was a path to follow to the world again. Teresa and I had talked weekly for two months; life was going on.

She told me about the miracle of cabbage for engorged breasts. It was discovered by some women in Australia. Chemists hadn't yet figured out what the active agent was, but something in cabbage stopped this powerful pain. JD lost no time getting to the store. I lined my bra with thick green leaves, feeling foolish and marveling at how the curves of the leaves were just right! The coolness felt good. In twenty minutes, the pain was gone. It was gone! About every two to four hours I had to change the leaves, but what bliss to have relief. The smell of coleslaw permeated the airspace. Something to laugh about was yet another gift. Friday night came, and we were almost through another day.

We decided to call and see how Mylah was doing. The phone call was hard to make. I didn't want to intrude. I needed to know how she was. My need was great; I didn't know if I could contain it in politeness. We called. Bear Cub was fine. She was eating, she was pooping regular poop now, no longer the sticky meconium. The trip back to Wisconsin was good. We kept the call brief.

I didn't sense the call was unwelcome, nor did I sense any compassion. Not one drop. I was totally happy for Alycia's joy, for the time of falling in love that was happening among the three of them. But I had heard story after story of adoptive parents crying, sharing the other side of their joy with the birth mom at the time of endings and beginnings. Where was that?

So far there had not been the word "thank-you" spoken. "Words cannot express what we feel," she had told the news reporter. But I needed words. The wall going up between us was going to be hard to live with.

I stayed clear in my self that what I did, this whole amazing adventure, I did for me. Without Alycia and Mandel, I would not have had this experience. I maintained my gratitude, feeling it deeply. My connection with Bear Cub was strong and good. I missed her fiercely, but the cord I had promised would stay was there. It was there. I didn't lose my joy or my pride in Mylah or the feeling of accomplishment. I worked at remembering the gratitude. These things saved me.

Saturday I made a trip to the grocery store for more cabbage, my new miracle drug. I walked around thinking I would be recognized from the many TV news spots, and feeling conspicuous. It was important to see that I was just one person on the planet, no matter the extraordinary events of the past days. I was just a person shopping for cabbage. The world was still there, like usual.

By Monday, I went to see Teresa to get some antibiotics to guard against mastitis and also an antiviral for the cold sore that was sprouting on my lip. I brought pictures to show the staff at Teresa's office. Most people brought in their babies to show.

I saw how much I was finding my own path through this experience, and how unsure people were about how to respond and what to say. Most everything anyone said was OK. The words that hurt were "Oh, the parents must be so thankful to you." And I tried not to say much, but just smile. I presented a happy face, talking about the good part, admitting, yes, it was hard. But there was a privacy to the hurt of missing Bear Cub that I wanted and needed to protect.

The first week was the worst. After that, other things began to fill into my life again. We planned a trip to Cozumel to bask in the sun. It was a wonderful trip. We celebrated JD's strong progress in his cancer fight and our successful trip throughout pregnancy and birthing. There, on a chance tour, we were taken to a Mayan ruin where women went after childbirth. It was the place not for birthing, but for giving thanks. I had been carrying a red hibiscus flower with me; I walked up onto the ancient square rock, I opened my heart to the tropical blue sky, and I held up my gratitude to the wind. Thanks for Bear Cub who now lives in and beyond my open heart. Thanks for the marvels of learning on the journey called pregnancy. Thanks for the courage in my heart and the power in the spirits of all people to do what we can to make life bigger. I left the flower red against the large grey stone.

For months there were few phone calls between our house and Alycia and Mandel's, none I didn't initiate. There was a letter and picture that came after Mylah was a month old. The news about her was wonderful. She was growing and learning and sleeping. She was a calm baby and vibrant and strong. No surprises to me. Alycia was heartbroken by having to return to work, and yet she did have to in order to make ends meet. I wrote back, expressing gratitude for the news, and empathy about the pain of needing to be away from one's baby.

JD and I visited first in March, spending a day at their house with Mylah, as her parents worked. Alycia was gracious to us. I didn't reach for Bear Cub, but waited to have her offered to me to hold. She looked different. A lifetime had passed. I felt awkward. I was monitoring my feelings before they were formed. But those first moments passed, and we settled into a good day.

Mylah was wonderful. I gave her a denim romper I had embroidered with a red heart, a bear cub, and a strong tall tree. I tied red suede slippers I had made on her cherished feet. She kicked them off every chance she got. She liked to swing. She liked me to sing to her. She smiled some, and made sounds with us. We reveled in her presence in the same way winter-weary folk turn themselves toward the spring sunshine. Then Mandel came home: It was time to say good-bye. And we did. The pain at parting was intense but not long lasting; a sign to me that there was honesty and progress in my grieving.

We arranged to have Mylah visit for several days in June. We asked for that privilege, and Alycia and Mandel needed child care to fill in a gap in their regular provider's schedule right then. It was a wonderful joy to bring her home and to take part in her care. She was familiar to me, and I was oddly comfortable taking care of a baby. Before, I had felt unsure.

After three days in South Dakota, we brought her back home to Wisconsin, and lay with her on a blanket on the front lawn of Alycia and Mandel's home. JD touched Mylah's face with a piece of feathery, blooming grass. She smiled at the touch. I smiled at his gentleness and her delight. Again, the parting was hard, and painful, and we passed through it back into our lives.

Learning to be in this family, this grouping of parents and child; learning to be in this precarious balancing of love and distance will take time. But, it can be learned.

The Gift of a Child

In many societies, the concepts of parent and child and the roles of mates are much more fluid than they are where I grew up in mainstream mid-America. Native Americans I knew used "cousin" in a way that extends far beyond a blood tie. And often one's "relations" extend to all creation—birds, rocks, and bison as well as Auntie Alice. In Native Hawaiian tradition one might have hānai children and hānai parents, an additional family often not related by blood. Those ideas significantly change the fabric of common life. Lives with more fluid understandings seem less tangled and more connected. In such societies, this story of surrogacy might not seem so unusual.

But for so many Western people, where relationships are built as if there is ownership involved, to "give away" a child is beyond reason. We "have" children and are married "to" someone. And in such relationships of owning, people become commodities. And we are not commodities, we know it from our early years on, and so we rip and tear at that fabric that enslaves. Yet, even when we break free, we so often weave the same tangled illusion back for ourselves as if control and being controlled is the only social fabric there is.

Obligation has replaced choice and generosity: A father is shackled to a lifelong job in order to provide for people he begins to ignore and grows to hate; a mother becomes a martyr and gives up her dreams, and so lights the twin fires of depression in herself and guilt in her children; children deny the parts of themselves their parents would not recognize, and limp along fifty years later blaming parents long dead. Mates, too, suffer massively when the illusion that we belong to each other fails. Are the promise and beauty of relating in love lost precisely because we relate to people as if they belong to us or we to them?

From the moment the Great Mystery rubs two cells together and strikes a spark, we belong first and finally to ourselves. That is the other way: living in the gentle power of humility, possessing one's self and no others; loving, then, with an open heart. Everything changes with that shift. Suddenly we are not married "to" but married "with" a partner. We do not "have" children, but "live with" children. Even our social institutions, educational models, and businesses would change. The destructive patterns of ownership are everywhere.

We need not live forever in debt to our parents. We need not hold them responsible for all that we need. Also, we are not duty bound to meet all our children's needs. And they are not meant to be our reason to live. That is not love.

A Wampanog man who was trying to return to the traditions and wisdom of his heritage once told me he needed to teach and offer guidance to his children carefully, because as children they were likely more whole in spirit than he. I watched him with his young son and daughter. It wasn't just a romantic idea from a less complicated time. He didn't dominate them. He fathered them when they needed it. They related as essentially equal. All of them had dignity. That is love. It is not an easy path, but it is rich.

I live now with Bear Cub as a presence in my life. And, I celebrate her being that extends so far beyond mine. I miss her. And I cherish her. I walk into my future on this new ground, on the many gifts I have been given by this child. Those truths take me ever away from suffering and entanglement and ever toward the healing wholeness of Home. All in all, what is lost is nothing compared to what is found.

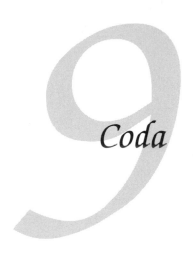

Coda

Two years and eight months after Mylah's birth Alycia and I met again. Beyond all odds, we found our way back to friendship.

Over the previous few months, our e-mails began carrying more than talk of Mylah, a few words of query about each other, an expression of concern, a personal affirmation or revelation. Our words contained spring winds. Between us, river ice snapped and cracked and heaved, breaking up our long winter. With more warm words there was water flowing again between the shores of my friend and me. Waters that flowed with the possibility of new life. We found ourselves with an option again. The option wasn't easy, but we each seemed to know that our friendship was now able to be coaxed out of hibernation.

I was ready to let go of what I assumed to be true in Alycia. I found myself ready to listen to what she had to say about this experience from her own passage through it. I was curious. I cared. I wanted to understand. Alycia was eager for healing too, for the reconnection of our friendship. We both reached out. We planned to meet for an extended visit, seeing each other several times over three weeks. Alycia scheduled a week off work and I made arrangements to fly to her town. In the previous year, both of our households moved to different states and the distance between us was now great. We would spend several of the daytimes together, just Alycia and I, trying to sort through it all. We would play together with Mylah in the evenings and enjoy time with Mandel over supper. I would go see other people and come back. Time apart, time together. Time for healing.

I arrived, checked into my hotel, and called Alycia. With a bravery I had missed seeing in Alycia for years, she knocked on my hotel door. We hugged. Across all the months and all the hurt, across all the difficult choices and the broken time, we hugged each other. For the first time since Mylah's birth, I greeted Alycia before I greeted Mylah. And then, with Mylah in the lead for the first day, the three of us played and talked and laughed, finding our way. That first afternoon was like clearing the land between us, overgrown as it was with caution, hurt, misunderstanding, neglect, weeds that choke out love and friendship.

Mylah was a delight to see. It had been over a year since our last visit. Mylah had grown from a baby to a toddler. Her command of language now made communicating with her immediate. No more guessing, now she said what she wanted and what was on her mind and in her heart. Her spirit, that powerful, joyful, loving presence I had known in the pregnancy, was there in full force. I was afraid each time I was about to see her that somehow I didn't have it right, that I had made her up, that she wasn't really the child I had imagined. But there she was, at the end of my long plane ride, and she was just who I knew and remembered. She was shy with me for a minute or two, then warmed and smiled and we were off for hours of playful adventure and fun. I spent the evening alone with Mylah because Alycia and Mandel had a dinner party to attend. I held her, read to her, touched her toes and hands, her face, her curls. I recognized the child who is so undoubtedly my daughter, and basked in her tangible presence.

During the next three days, Alycia and I talked together without Mylah. It took great courage to ask the questions, to answer them, to surface the pain that was festering. We each had thorns embedded deep inside that needed extracting. We had the time, we each were willing. But courage is never easy to find. We began with some clumsy confessions to get the shadows of our guilt off of our hearts. Alycia expressed her grief that she hadn't been able to move through the pregnancy and birthing in the way that felt right to her. She knew she hadn't done her best. We cried and held each other. I said I had expected many things from her that were too much to ask, that I saw in her eyes now that I had wanted her to do and be what she could not do or be. I was wrong to do that. The barriers between us were made by each of us, and our initial confessions opened the locks on the doors.

Where was the courage we needed to approach each other? How would we find our way? The day before, we walked down the hotel hallway with Mylah in the middle, holding each of our hands. Unprompted, Mylah looked up to me and said, "You're my other mommy!"

I said, "Yes I am."

She turned to Alycia, "You're my mommy," and turning to me again, "and you're my other mommy." She smiled widely at each of us, and laughed.

My heart jumped and danced when she called me Mommy. Alycia and I, after responding to Mylah's wide smiling heart, looked into each other's faces. We knew that no matter how hard it would be to untangle the threads of love and friendship between us, we would do it. This child holding each of our hands deserved the best we could offer her. She called the best out of us. She gave us the gift of a vision of the simple truth. She said so simply, "You're my mommy and you're my other mommy." We needed to face what that truth meant in all its adult complexities.

Sitting together, set apart from all distraction, Alycia and I gathered our resolve, we set our faces to look at everything we needed to see. We joined our hands. We would not let go until we did what we could do to bring healing to each of us and to our friendship. We would use the manuscript of this book, and read through it word by word together, stopping our reading when we needed to ask, to listen, to clarify, to question, or to cry.

Near the beginning of our talking, I asked her to tell me what had been happening to her since the pregnancy—overall, how she was making sense of this time. She struggled. Her words were faltering. She couldn't express in words what was inside of her. Alycia is a painter, a visual artistic soul. So I suggested she use images instead of words to describe a visual representation of her experience. She quickly gathered all the feelings into an image. The whole complex image flowed out of her like watercolors onto a canvas.

Before all this, she told me, she had been an iron bar, rectangular and strong, mighty, resistant to tension. That strength served her well in many difficult battles in her life. She trusted it. But going through this pregnancy and birth and becoming a mother had changed her fundamentally.

The Gift of a Child

The iron bar of her self was heated from the inside. It began to heat from the hurt, the anger, the frustration of her infertility, of all the emotions of our pregnancy and our broken relationship, from the cultural expectations, from factors she could not even identify. The iron bar glowed inside, and the heat spread outward. Her trusted protection heated inside of her to red hot, to pliability. And then those outside forces pummeled her, pounded her. Those forces were the injustice of not being able to conceive, the raw fact of her infertility, the specific manifestation of being unable to create life, a child, with her beloved Mandel. Her iron rod self was beaten on by the way the world was. Pounded by how I could conceive and she couldn't. Pounded by family and societal expectations that she become a mother. Like a farrier beats a red-hot horseshoe, she was shaped and ultimately opened up and spread out until the bar of metal was flat and circular.

Then, before having any time to adjust or recalibrate her own changed shape, she was drowned by this experience. In the midst of her pain she was plunged down into the water, hot metal hissing as it cooled. And then, she was left alone to learn who she was again.

First, she was aware of her anger. She roared from having been distorted, misshapen, weakened, and so fundamentally exposed. Her strength itself had been altered.

Many months came and went. In that time she grew to know herself as Mylah's mother. And gradually Alycia learned different names for what had happened for her. She wasn't disfigured and distorted, but metamorphosed, transfigured. She wasn't weakened, but perfected. On this day, as we talked together in my hotel room lying on the huge king-sized bed, she was open for a new picture of her strength. She saw herself now as a copper bowl, blackened in spots, burnished. Not smooth, but dented. The beating and pounding on her spirit had created beauty, meaning, patterns, and designs in this bowl of her strength. This was now who she was. Someone new.

The telling of this extended image came to completion. She breathed deeply. That is how the experience had been for her. She communicated the years of trial to me well. I felt her breath, her fingerprint, her heartbeat in these images. I respected the enormity of her transformation. What I had seen from the outside of her was not at all what had been happening for her. And now, with utter honesty, she had shown me where she had been.

I hesitated to speak. There was a picture in my mind as she described the copper bowl. After there had been quiet for a time, I told her I had seen that rustic, beautiful bowl. I had seen her sitting cross-legged, with Mylah resting in the bowl of her body, cradled against her as they had read books together the afternoon before. Alycia's eyes deepened. She saw what I was describing.

I felt cautious to touch the new image so central to her, but the image was full of energy. Was, perhaps, this transformation from the iron rod to the copper bowl because Mylah needed a mother who knew what Alycia now knew? Maybe Mylah needed a mother who had learned the painfully potent lessons she had been taught. Alycia sat up and grabbed onto what I was saying. She immediately said it was true. The energy flowed through her. She knew that, from this moment on, what had felt like a barrage of unwelcome attacks could be seen as a series of profound gifts. Painful. Unchosen. But they were gifts given to turn her into a mother. She said she knew intuitively that if all the pain had been required of her in order to have the gift of raising Mylah, she would have volunteered for it. Some enormous pall lifted off of her, and months and years of pain were released. Gratitude itself transforms.

Spiritual pregnancy. Spiritual labor. Her changes were not physical. Her pain was not in her muscles and nerves. But Alycia knows pregnancy and labor in its truest form: being challenged beyond your ability, being forced to trust a side of yourself you do not know is trustworthy, forever leaving behind a comfortable land for one that is wholly new. She endured the deepest forms of pregnancy and labor, and reemerged in gratitude. The capacity for human beings to persevere during physical and emotional pain is greatly increased when there is a reason, a result, something that is learned.

We talked further about these insights, about labor, about our different schooling through our different pregnancies. Still full from articulating what had been happening for her, Alycia said, "The experience was not what we thought it would be." After some thought she added, "It was not what we wanted it to be." She paused quite a while. "It was perfect." Her eyes deepened again. Our talking quieted. She lay back down. We were like mirror images of each other. We breathed into a silence of truth alone. "Why is it so difficult for us to imagine the best?" she whispered to me. I held the question with her. She answered herself, "Because, the best is the hardest." Her courage and truth brought rain to the drought in her soul and we laughed and cried.

The healing brought us to deeper layers of truth. I began to understand how much I had underestimated the depth and complexity of how it was for Alycia to live on with the wound of her infertility. Over the years, her confidence had eroded. By the time we conceived, she felt compelled to primally protect her self and the scraps of hope she still held in her fist. She clutched onto her hope for a child, keeping it compressed and small. She could not let that hope blossom. Especially if it was outside of her own self, her own control. She was instinct driven, and felt if this hope was dashed, she would die. She would die.

I did not understand that it had cost Alycia everything to act out her hope for a child with others involved, to say yes to this process, to consent to the conception. It would be like a person who was dying of thirst agreeing to allow someone else to carry her the only cup of water there was. She agreed. But then was spent.

She had no trust to invest in me. It wasn't that she perceived me as untrustworthy, she simply had no trust left. She had spent her trust repeatedly placing her hope in the goodness of the universe, the Giver she felt would provide her a child. Now, pushed past trust, she wasn't merely angry or hurt or jealous that I had conceived and she hadn't. She was catapulted into an unknown land by that fact. A land for which she had no maps. Our conception was easy to achieve. What was God saying to her in this event? Why did it take four people for her to have a baby? Reality shifted, reorganized all around her. Trust? She knew only she might die. She was risking everything. And in order to have her dream she indeed lost most of who she thought she was, and much of what she imagined her dream to be.

Alycia's sister offered her a gift as the pregnancy progressed, a pendant of a woman with a round stone belly.

It was to be a sign of Alycia's own pregnancy. Alycia loved it. But it also became for her a tortured symbol of the way she was and wasn't pregnant. At times, when waiting through our gestation, Alycia admitted, she pretended she was pregnant. But what she thought might be a way of entering into joy became a source of terrible pain. And though she knew she was indeed pregnant in some mysterious way, still that boundary between mystery and make-believe was illusive. She couldn't afford the shock of unexpected locked doors, the slam to her body of a stairway she thought had one more step. She gave up believing in the mystery that was real because she couldn't endure the shock of the locked door when she wasn't expecting it. The little pendant, given in pure love, now held all the tortured freight of infertility.

For Alycia, to be a mother was not something that could involve someone else. She was confused, as I was, with my feeling like a mother when the pregnancy began to take root. In her mind there couldn't be two mothers with one baby, and so she backed away; she submerged her own budding mother feelings, submitting to me. She tucked herself under me, not standing up beside me as I was wanting.

What I felt as lack of support, she saw as a way of being out of my way. In the tangles of her unconscious she felt her inability to conceive and attain pregnancy infected her, and that her closeness to me might taint our pregnancy. She saw her presence as potentially damaging, and withheld words, questions, her thoughts, indeed her friendship with the intention of protecting me from her own infertile self.

Truth heals. Knowing and speaking and hearing honest truth heals deeply. Hearing what had been true for her unhooked the hurts in me. They simply were carried off down that once-frozen river between us. Forgiveness as an act of will wasn't necessary. When we understood each other, the hurts were knots untied; they were no more. As we talked on and on, we found this kind of unfiltered honesty bringing us together. What a surprise. Even though we were sharing the extinguished flames of our angers with each other, we were growing in love.

I talked with her about my feelings of being abandoned by her, neglected, left alone in our joint pregnancy. I risked sharing, not every little issue, but the core of that feeling. Alycia listened, the feelings I expressed registered on her face. She knew what I was talking about. And she knew why it had happened.

Alycia rearranged herself, sitting near me, and told me another astonishing secret. She had not wanted to share this pregnancy. She had not wanted to have a child this way. She had been, in a sense, forced into making this choice by her infertility, and felt cheated out of an experience she desperately wanted. What I had named and experienced as acts and expressions of neglect were, again, much more. It was not nearly so personal. She was refusing to participate any more than she absolutely had to in my pregnancy. My pregnancy that meant she was not pregnant. It made all the sense in the world, but I had never considered it.

She had not wanted to share this pregnancy with me. And with new understanding, I remembered my feeling of being an intruder as she sang the lullaby to my newly pregnant belly, her distance from me, and what I saw as her lack of interest in the pregnancy. She hadn't wanted to share it. And so she didn't. And so in many ways, she cut herself off from what she might have experienced of Mylah's beginnings.

And still, she couldn't hate me or focus her anger and hurt on me consciously. I was the evidence of her failure, and also the doorway through which her hope would fly into her life. With a stranger, perhaps, the feelings of being cheated could have been easily projected onto a surrogate, but for Alycia, the complexity was unending. The layers of emotion, the multiplicity of roles, the sources of pain and hope all made the pregnancy a very confusing time. A swirling of essences. She stilled in the midst of it, grew silent from a desire not to intensify the brokenness, not to inflict more damage.

It seems in my life I need to learn over and over that I do not understand more than a whiff of what is happening for any other person.

Convinced now that I understood so little of what we had been through, I sought to unravel all that was not true. I raised the issue of what I had seen as a lack of interest in bonding with the child forming in my body, the lack of interest in reading to her or acknowledging her, in cuddling with her the best we could after seeing those first ultrasound pictures. After expressing my question, I looked into Alycia's face. Her eyes were clear, her face naked. There was the truth I had not been able to imagine. At that moment it seemed clear. Embarrassingly clear. How could she have begun to bond, or even truly acknowledged the baby, and then driven away home again and lived her childless life? I felt a chill of identification. I knew the pain of walking away and of being left without Mylah. I had factored it in from the beginning. I had chosen it. It was something for which I was prepared. How could she have born that tearing of souls, the distance, before ever even knowing the touch of the little one, her scent, her kick. Looking at her face, I saw that bearing the distance between mother and daughter isn't possible if one hasn't first had the intimate time. I felt foolish. Alycia reassured me. We didn't know. We just didn't know what we had each been experiencing. This moment also confirmed for me my decision to have time to say hello to Mylah before being asked to say good-bye.

I asked even more. The trips to visit often were canceled and difficult to plan, how did that fit in? She took a deep breath, nodding her head up and down. She knew. Even more than Alycia, Mandel had difficulty sharing what he wanted to be happening inside their marriage, inside Alycia's body. Alycia suspected that for Mandel to see my belly full of their child would have been incongruous. He is a man who does not express himself easily in words. Much happened for him beneath the surface of nouns and verbs, in the land of decisions and actions. He changed his mind about visits. There were always other things he needed to be doing. He was protecting the boundary of what he could deal with.

Alycia somehow sensed to be all five together with my pregnancy large and evident would be too much for Mandel to bear. She rightly needed to maintain her connection with him, their unity as a couple. For Mandel, the intrusion that I was perceived to be was too difficult to process without words. The illusion of adultery was perhaps also a complicating factor. For him, the confusion of realities was perhaps the most difficult. And so, Alycia needed to follow his lead, and where he was not able to lead them, she could not travel.

As the sharing and thorn pulling progressed between Alycia and me, understanding grew between us. What had been confusing was now fitting into place. As the questions were asked and answers and information shared from the painful broken time, Alycia and I found the ease of communication returning to us that we each had treasured for so many years. Neither of us had any other woman with whom we could truly share the depth of what it had been like to go through this surrogacy experience. To find each other again, the only other one on the planet who could exactly understand, was a gift we thought might have been gone forever.

Alycia read the part of the manuscript about Mylah's birth in silence. She read every word. It was for her as if she had been finally admitted to the room where Mylah was born. She seemed wholly focused on getting to the place where Mylah emerged, where Alycia could "hear" Mylah's first breath. She said she finally didn't feel excluded anymore. Finally, she had some sense of witnessing Mylah's birth. But what the birthing had been like for me didn't seem to be of much interest to her.

Alycia didn't talk much about it all, slowly absorbing what she had been so hungry for. When she arrived at the part in the story where she and Mandel burst into the room and she saw Mylah for the first time, her voice returned. Mylah was bundled up, in the car seat, ready to make the wintery trip to our house. Alycia told me she wanted to take off all the baby's clothes, to see her, all of her, and to meet her naked as she was born. Once more the distance separated her and her dream, this time the distance of mere fabric. And this time, after one more dear day, this perfect whole child would be in her care.

We spent time remembering the day after Mylah was born, when Alycia and Mandel came to pick her up and bring her to their home. Alycia said she did have compassion that day. She saw agony in my eyes, in my armored self. She imagined her way inside my agony, imagined the tearing apart, the dismemberment of having my child leave me; and she couldn't bear to wound me so. She couldn't leave our house that day because she couldn't make this separation between me and Mylah happen. Courage. It is something that requires us to be many things that we would rather not need to be. She had to find the courage to do what she knew she needed to do. It was all underneath the casual words and the frosting faces, but she knew, she knew. The amount of courage required by each of the five of us that day was beyond measure. I could not respect her surface laughter. But, I could respect her need to gather courage.

I spoke of my emptiness, and of the deepest part of that painful separating: that I didn't know that I would ever see Mylah again until she was of age to choose to see me. I wasn't sure, given how things were between the four of us, that there would be any relationship between me and my daughter. Alycia listened. She took in the truth of that horrifying statement. She said, "Do you know about Mylah's name?"

And in my remembered grief there was a birdsong. I had wanted, beyond all reason, to have some connection to Mylah's name, to have a tie with her in that public and personal place of her name. And still I knew that could only be given to me, not requested by me. And here I was, hoping against hope that she would tell me a story that might heal this broken-winged hope. I looked into Alycia's face, this time my vulnerability was on display.

First she had to admit something she said was a nasty thing. She hadn't told me this story earlier because she wanted to keep the meaning of Mylah's name secret from me, to balance in some small way the power and the control I had in so many ways. "Good for you!" I said. We laughed. I have always identified with rebellion, the spirited standing up for one's self, sometimes in unnoticeable, subtle ways. Those acts of self-assertion in impossible situations keep people afloat in stormy seas.

She had chosen a name that started with "M" because both Mandel and Mary Ann did. The name "Mylah" was suggested by her sister. Alycia decided that beside the "M" there was a "Y" from Alycia and Mary Ann; an "L" from Alycia; an "A" from Mandel, Alycia, and Mary Ann; and an "H" that was all Mylah's own. Alycia didn't know what JD's initials stood for, but chose

Darrelle for a middle name. Darrell was the name JD was known by as a boy. He is John Darrell. We knew late in the pregnancy that "Darrelle" and "Mylah" were names they were considering. So I knew this amazing coincidence with Darrelle before Mylah's birth. But the reason for "Mylah," the meanings of the letters, Alycia kept, appropriately, to herself until this marathon of secret telling and healing.

Mylah's name had a connection to me. I was overwhelmed. I told Alycia that at the birth I was desperate to feel some ongoing connection with my daughter, some assurances that the tie we had was recognized and respected by the world, but mostly by Alycia. Now, here was the gift, as wonderful as I had hoped for. The grace we needed, even though we could not always fully express it to each other, the grace was given to us. We had it to share.

As we talked, it became clear to us both that all through the struggles of the broken time, we did have all we needed in order to have a loving and positive experience. We just didn't always share it. If the four of us put the truths of our emotions and beliefs into a bucket; and if we each took out of that bucket what we needed to have, there would have been enough for every need.

Seeing this helped both Alycia and me restore some of our faith. As people raised in Christianity, we each had been taught that underneath are the everlasting arms, that somehow, through whatever comes, there is a circle of love around us. We are not guaranteed safety, but we are guaranteed that we need never be alone. We are guaranteed love. That is a treasure I have tested many times and found to be true.

But, during this emotional and spiritual climb up the Mt. Everest of this surrogacy experience, each of the four of us in our own way questioned the presence of those arms. Perhaps all people come to that questioning in their lives. There comes a time when the Presence isn't perceived. If we had each acted out of our courage every time, if we had been able to offer the best we had inside of us every moment to the others in our tiny circle of four, there was given to us what each one needed. That insight restores my faith. The lesson is always, no matter how difficult it seems, to give what I have to give, to be all of my best self.

There is another related but almost opposite lesson I also learned. Alycia and I were often looking for the other one to meet our needs. I wanted Alycia to support me more. She wanted me to communicate more. I wanted her to see me as I was, a woman pregnant, a woman releasing her child to another woman. Alycia wanted me to recognize the enormous sacrifice she had already made, the total relinquishing of her own dream, and to give her all that she was needing. As we talked that day two and a half years later, we saw that in nearly every circumstance, the gifts we were looking for in each other we already had in ourselves.

We are unaccustomed to meeting our own profound needs, of seeing our own selves as vehicles the Holy One uses to support us. And yet, in some circumstances, that is precisely the way our needs are best met. In putting the locus of the "solution" to our pain outside ourselves, Alycia and I blinded ourselves to what was being given to us. As we came together for this week of reconnecting and sifting, sorting through the story, we each heard, most often in our own words and our own insights, all we needed to be whole. First, and finally, we belong to ourselves, and it is often we who can best meet our own deep needs.

In between all the emotion wrangling, 2½-year-old Mylah sat with Alycia and me on their kitchen floor after pulling out the cooking pots and bowls she uses in play. The talk and intensity of the day had depleted us. Alycia and I were eager to just play with Mylah. And there she sat, cooking up an invisible batch of supper for us. She scooped up big bowls of her mysterious dinner, and we all ate. We played, and still it wasn't just pretend. She fed us. She always has been a teacher, from the moment of her conception.

One evening, when Mandel came home, Mylah ran to the door to greet him, then took him by the hand, insistently leading him to where I was. She put his hand

and my hand together. "Hug," she said. "Hug." She looked back and forth between us with her solemn face, and waited. And so Mandel and I hugged. We were each more interested in her, perhaps than each other, but we did hug. In many ways we did begin reweaving a friendship. I didn't feel the need to sort things through with Mandel, to repair damage, to explore the meanings of all that had happened. We just moved on. And the hug was a sign we were beginning to do that for Mylah.

A different day, as Alycia and I were playing with Mylah on the floor, Mylah made our toes touch on one side of her. As our bodies curved around on opposite sides of her, she joined our hands, and sat beaming and laughing inside the circle of her two mommies.

This was a visit I needed to make on my own, and still there were many moments we all missed JD being there with us. I talked a little about JD to Mylah. I showed her some pictures of Baby Mylah with me and JD. But when I called JD, she didn't want to talk with him on the phone. I was feeling sad for him to be missing out on this reunion. Then in the car one day as we all were heading out to lunch after visiting a petting zoo, Mylah said something I didn't understand. Alycia turned around and asked her again what she said. "My other daddy is JD." Her pronunciation wasn't exact but that is what she said, wholly unprompted. How she put together the pieces, I do not know. That evening we quickly sent an account of the story to JD, and it more than made up for her lack of interest in talking with him on the phone. He is sure of their bond, and feels sure that renewing his connection with Mylah will happen in its own time.

At bedtime one night she made her awareness of her own identity most clear. She gave her baby doll, wrapped in her special soft green blanket, to Alycia to hold. Then Mylah's sweet face looked up at me. She saw my arms empty, and looked worried. "You want a baby too?" her girl voice clear and true as her blue eyes.

"Oh," I said, "we can share."

She became quiet, very thoughtful, and then went to Alycia. "Your turn is up." She gently took the baby from Alycia's arms, brought it over to me. "Now it's your turn." Over the course of the evening play and story reading, Mylah carried the baby doll back and forth between us, saying, "Your turn is up. Now it's your turn," smiling wildly at our stunned reaction to her.

Awe. Nothing less than awe that in a 2½-year-old way, she comprehends the mysterious, joyous circumstance of her coming to birth.

For Alycia as for me, Mylah is clearly a child who belongs to herself. A little whole person whose life is her very own. In the heart of our hearts we are not jealous of the love, the mother bonds, the unique ways we each have attachments to this little girl. It is so clear to me that Alycia is Mylah's perfect mother. I wouldn't want less for Mylah. And though it took me days to trust it, Alycia is clearly delighted in the strong bond between Mylah and me.

Our friends do not seem to understand this. Many people encourage Alycia to cut off the friendship with me out of fear that I will somehow endanger her bond with Mylah. Some say I am interfering when I keep in touch with Mylah. People seem not to believe that I don't want to be raising this child I love, and that I recognize Alycia as the best mother Mylah could have. They think I am just making that up to appease my own loss. It isn't true. Love doesn't require possessiveness. Alycia has what she wants and needs with Mylah. I have what I want and need with Mylah. We are not threats to each other. In the heart of things, love is much stronger than possession. I am perhaps first in the line of those who would defend Alycia as Mylah's mother. And Alycia is first in the line of those who would defend me as Mylah's mother. Mylah is not a possession. I did not give her away. She belongs, as we all do, to herself.

Alycia and I are as astounded as anyone that this is how it actually is. But we truly are finding the only way to move comfortably ahead is on this path of openness and love. The deep truths within us are not in conflict. There is no need for jealousy. We are living, to the shock of many, a life based on open-hearted love. The one who is not surprised is Mylah.

The grace of being a mother to Mylah is one of the richest honors either of us has ever experienced. I hope the learning that comes to the five of us through the years of this shared family life continues and continues. I hope this most difficult adventure never ends.

Inner Ocean Publishing publishes in the genres of self-help, personal growth, lifestyle, conscious business, and inspirational nonfiction. Our goal is to publish books that touch the spirit and make a tangible difference in the lives of individuals, families, and their communities.

The six books in our Fall 2002 list reflect our company's goals, depict the process of personal growth and spiritual exploration that we cultivate in ourselves and others, and encourage a sense of personal responsibility in our individual, business, and global affairs. We invite you to visit us at:
www.innerocean.com.
Aloha.

Mystical Dogs:
Animals as Guides to Our Inner Life
Jean Houston

In the High-Energy Zone:
The 6 Characteristics of Highly Effective Groups
Paul Deslauriers

Sacred Selfishness:
A Guide to Living a Life of Substance
Bud Harris, Ph.D.

Universal Water:
The Ancient Wisdom and Scientific Theory of Water
West Marrin, Ph.D.

Choosing to Be Well:
A Conscious Approach to a Healthier Lifestyle
Haven Logan, Ph.D.

The Gift of a Child
Mary Ann Thompson